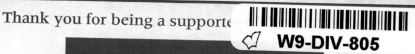

Thank you for being a supporte

HOD
Halachic Organ Donor
S O C I E T Y

www.hods.org   212-213-5087   admin@hods.org

THE ETHICS OF TRANSPLANTS

THE ETHICS OF
TRANSPLANTS

Why Careless Thought Costs Lives

JANET RADCLIFFE RICHARDS

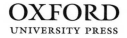

OXFORD

UNIVERSITY PRESS

OXFORD
UNIVERSITY PRESS

Great Clarendon Street, Oxford OX2 6DP

Oxford University Press is a department of the University of Oxford.
It furthers the University's objective of excellence in research, scholarship,
and education by publishing worldwide in

Oxford New York

Auckland Cape Town Dar es Salaam Hong Kong Karachi
Kuala Lumpur Madrid Melbourne Mexico City Nairobi
New Delhi Shanghai Taipei Toronto

With offices in

Argentina Austria Brazil Chile Czech Republic France Greece
Guatemala Hungary Italy Japan Poland Portugal Singapore
South Korea Switzerland Thailand Turkey Ukraine Vietnam

Oxford is a registered trade mark of Oxford University Press
in the UK and in certain other countries

Published in the United States
by Oxford University Press Inc., New York

British Library Cataloguing in Publication Data
Data available

Library of Congress Cataloging in Publication Data
Data available

Typeset by SPI Publisher Services, Pondicherry, India
Printed in Great Britain
on acid-free paper by
Clays Ltd., St Ives plc

ISBN 978–0–19–957555–8

1

As this book was in the final stage of production we heard that David Price, whom I acknowledge in the Preface, had died on 3 January 2012.

The news of his illness, only a couple of months earlier, had come as a deep shock to all his colleagues. He was a lovely man: one of those rare people whom everyone regarded with affection as well as respect. He once remarked that the people who seemed most pleased to see him were grandchildren and dogs, but I hope he realized that even if the rest of us were less frisky in our demonstrations of enthusiasm, everybody was delighted by any meeting with him. We will miss him acutely.

This book is dedicated to the memory of David Price.

PREFACE

The work that led to this book began by accident in the early 1990s, as the result of a brief flirtation I had with journalism. During that period there erupted a scandal about Turkish peasants who had come to London as paid kidney donors, and it was an obvious subject for an article. Most journalism sinks without trace, but this piece happened to be picked up by a transplant surgeon—Robert Sells, of the Liverpool Royal Infirmary—who was deeply concerned about the matter, and who invited me to speak at an innovative international conference on transplant ethics in Munich, in 1992. I was impressed by his invitation, because he knew, from the article, that I would be arguing against his own position. This suggested that he was more concerned to get to the root of the problems than to defend his own intuitions; and at the Munich meeting it became clear that many other professionals in the field were beginning to realize the extent and depth of the moral problems raised by the developments in transplantation, and of the need for serious interdisciplinary work.

Since that time I have found it impossible to drop the subject, even though it was not, and in a way still is not, central to my academic work. Soon afterwards I became part of the International

Forum for Transplant Ethics, a small group that Professor Sells and a few colleagues—including such highly distinguished ones as Sir Raymond Hoffenberg and Sir (now but not then) Ian Kennedy— were setting up for the purpose of questioning all the currently received wisdom in the area. That involvement, as well as requests for conference contributions, lectures, papers, and book chapters, has kept the subject simmering in the background of my work ever since, to the extent that I suspect most people in the transplant field think I do nothing else. This book itself began as an attempt to pull together the bits and pieces that had accumulated in obscure publications over the years, and get the whole thing out of the way— though I somehow doubt that that will happen. Apart from anything else, I have still nowhere near finished my own thinking about it. Practical moral philosophy is an extraordinarily difficult subject, and every step of the enquiry throws up new complications.

What got me going in the first place, and led me to choose the subject of organ selling—or paid donation—for one of my journalistic experiments, was not so much the topic itself as the hopeless confusion of the arguments in the public debate. There were passionate feelings about the matter, and these led rapidly to statements of denunciation by associations of transplant professionals, and to legislation outlawing any payment for organ donation. But the arguments that were being used to justify these policies could have been used to illustrate basic mistakes in argument for undergraduate classes in informal logic. In fact I have often used them since for just this purpose. I did not, and do not, agree with the conclusion that payment should be universally prohibited; but the reason for this non-standard opinion is not that I came to the debate with radically different moral feelings from the people who reached the opposite conclusion, let alone any specialist knowledge of facts that undermined their claims. It was just that the principles being invoked as the basis of the political conclusions simply did not support the conclusions they were supposed to support, or were incompatible with principles regularly used by the same people in other contexts, or both.

Since I kept being invited to give lectures on the subject of payment, I used the opportunities to work on developing principles of moral reasoning relevant to all debates about policy: techniques of analysis that can be applied to any area of practical ethics, including others in the transplant field. The resulting enquiry has led me to several conclusions that I certainly was not expecting when I started pulling the work together for this book. Moral enquiry starts, like much scientific enquiry, with intuitions that need to be tested, and while some of those intuitions stand up to scrutiny others do not, and the enquiries themselves keep leading to questions that do not even arise until others have been answered. New questions are still coming up, and the book is being published now not because I have finished it, but because I probably never will and I need to move on. Anyway, my editor is putting her foot down.

The book can be read in two ways: both as an analysis of transplant ethics itself and as a contribution to the methodology of moral reasoning in practical contexts. In its second capacity, I hope it will demonstrate that basic philosophical analysis is absolutely indispensable in debates about practical ethics. All practical decision making, at both clinical and political levels, will of course depend heavily on the facts, and therefore on the expertise of clinical and social experts in the field, but mistakes in moral reasoning have effects as significant as ignorance and mistakes about matters of fact. This topic, like all other parts of practical ethics, really does call for genuinely interdisciplinary cooperation.

I am not very good at letting people see drafts in progress, and as a result I have had little in the way of direct comments on the text. However, my excellent OUP editor, Latha Menon, managed by various subterfuges to get unfinished drafts to two experts in the field: David Price, Professor of Law at De Montfort University, who has a knowledge and expertise I wish I had, and Chris Rudge, formerly a transplant surgeon and for some time now head of UK Transplant, the government body responsible for organizing and trying to regulate this impossible area. I am immensely grateful to both of these distinguished colleagues for taking the time to read that early draft, and for their comments and advice. I hope I have dealt with the points they raised, but the book has changed a good deal since they read it, so they are not to be blamed if more problems have since appeared. I am also grateful to my husband, Derek Parfit, for reading the later drafts and giving me many detailed comments on the text. And finally, very many thanks to Latha Menon. It is thanks to her that the book is being published only a year later than originally intended. But for her subtle methods of cajoling and prodding and working on the psychology of deadlines, the book would still be a mountain of semi-sorted material a dozen times as long as the present slim volume. She is also a wonderful critic, and has given me a great deal of encouragement and advice.

Very many thanks to all these people, as also to the many transplant colleagues with whom I have been debating many of these matters for years. I wonder what they will make of the result. Unless I am banished from further congresses for heresy, which is not impossible, I may soon find out.

CONTENTS

I

INTRODUCTION

An inevitable tension

Everyone knows by now that transplantation is one of the marvels of twentieth-century medicine. If you are unlucky enough to find yourself with severe kidney or liver disease, or a defective heart or lungs, or even a ravaged face or missing arm—and you are also rich enough, or in a rich enough country—there are now chances of remedy that not long ago would have been out of the question. There also seems to be no stopping its progress. Hardly a month goes past without our hearing of some new achievement. As I was writing this chapter, a woman who had been given the first transplanted voice box spoke for the first time; as I was finishing the book, surgeons were preparing to transplant a womb from a mother to her daughter.

Like all such successes, these advances generate problems of their own. The more we can do, the more decisions we have to make about what we ought to do. Demands for medical treatment are endless, and even within rich countries we are confronting increasingly difficult questions about how to allocate limited resources, and whether marginal improvements in health or life expectancy are worth their escalating costs, and which risks we should take with innovative treatments. On a global scale, all such problems of affluence may themselves seem like expensive luxuries. But quite apart from all these familiar issues, the progress in science and technology keeps throwing up problems of entirely new kinds, by breaking down familiar categories of thought. We have, for instance, long-standing principles about medical confidentiality; but how should we interpret those now that our understanding of genetics means that keeping the confidence of one person means depriving relatives of knowledge of their own genetic make-up? We have traditions about the organization and legal rights of families, but what should we do about those traditions now that artificial reproduction is mixing biological, gestatory, and social parentage? Problems like these are not just of scale or degree, but of kind. The world has changed.

The ability to move functioning organs from one person to another is, historically speaking, a totally new phenomenon. From the point of view of the patient, transplantation may be just another remarkable life-saving or health-restoring treatment; but it is quite unlike others in that any organ put into one person must first be taken from somebody else. For every transplant recipient there must be a donor—or *source*, to use a neutral term—and the distinctive ethical and political problems of transplantation, as opposed to the ones it shares with most other parts of advanced medicine, are all connected with the matter of where the organs come from. This is the moral and intellectual core of transplantation ethics.

To put the matter objectively and starkly, there is a perpetual competition between the people who need organs and the rest of us who have them. We are all now potential sources of spare parts for people whose own organs have failed, and whose hope lies in getting one of ours. This means, for instance, that the people on the waiting list for transplants from deceased donors are, in effect, hoping that one of the rest of us will die so that they can have our organs. And, furthermore, their hopes are not for the incidental scraps left behind by those of us who have reached the inevitable end of a long life, because if we die from the wearing out of our own body parts they will not be of much use to anyone else. What the patients hoping for transplants need, ideally, is the sudden death of a young and healthy person, whose organs are still in good condition. If you need a new liver, you really want something like the liver of a young, abstemious man who has died in a motorcycle accident. If you are longing for a heart that will save the life of your newborn baby, the only thing that can provide what you need is the death of someone else's baby.

This does not mean that patients and their friends and families and medical teams are actively thinking of the matter in these terms. This is not meant as a description of anyone's state of mind. Patients are probably not thinking at all about the details of where the hoped-for organs will come from, let alone campaigning for the repeal of crash-helmet and seat-belt legislation to increase the number of available donors. There is no overt warfare between the patients' advocates and the public at large. In most cases all that is being asked for is the use of organs that would otherwise be wasted, and it is easy to be wholly in sympathy with that ambition. Still, the tension is inherent in the situation, and inevitably there are contexts where it gets close to the surface.

If you have serious renal disease, for instance, it is now well known that kidneys for transplant can be taken from living donors. This means that although you are not necessarily depending on the hope of someone else's death, the question must immediately arise among your family and friends of whether one of them should volunteer. In many cases there may be a suitable and wholly willing donor, but there is always the possibility of moral bullying, or direct bullying, or attempts at bribery or emotional deception, by or on behalf of the person who needs the transplant. And even when there is no hint of any such thing, there may well be feelings of guilt and discomfort among people who think they really ought to be offering to step in. The very fact that someone needs what you might in principle give—and for whom the gain would be much greater than the loss to you—may be enough to put strain in the air.

Again, if a dying patient is identified as a suitable donor, a transplant team hoping for donation has the difficult job of approaching the family with a request for consent. Even where this is not legally necessary, because the potential donor is on the transplant register, clinicians will not usually go ahead unless the family agrees. This has to be done quickly if preparations are to be made to keep the organs in a viable state, and such interruptions to the process of dying and bereavement are by all convention jarring and inappropriate, even when not profoundly distressing. Friends and relations should be able to concentrate entirely on the person who is dying, without distraction from vultures hovering around to swoop on the body and whisk it off to be disembowelled. Transplant coordinators are well trained, but approaching distraught relatives in this way is not a thing anyone enjoys doing, or that any close relative or friend can be expected to feel comfortable about. However conscientiously green a recycler you may be, it is difficult to regard someone close to you, who has suddenly and probably traumatically died, as an inanimate store of replacement parts for someone else.

Behind the scenes, too, there is inevitable scope for discomfort, often (though by no means always) realized in practice. On the one hand there are the intensive care professionals, doing all they can to keep seriously ill or injured patients alive and interacting all the time with their distressed families, while on the other there are the transplant professionals who are equally anxious, on behalf of their own sick and dying patients, not to miss any opportunity to use the organs of patients who do die. This is probably the only context in which the failure of one group of doctors to save their patients is a necessary condition of another group's saving theirs. It is hardly surprising if mutterings occasionally surface from transplanters who suspect intensive care professionals of letting potential donors slip through their fingers, or from intensivists resentful of the surgeons who descend to ransack their dead patients and disappear to life-saving glory, leaving the colleagues on whom their work depends to cope with the mess and grief that remain.

The fact that transplant medicine can succeed only by means of giving one person the organs that some other person would ideally have preferred to keep has, not surprisingly, an enormous effect on the public perception of transplantation. In most parts of medicine sympathy is directed towards patients who cannot get the treatment they need, and in countries where the state has undertaken to provide health care for everyone there will often be public anger when resources are not made available. When journalists can show that people are being denied expensive treatment that might delay death from cancer by even a few months, for instance, or that has some statistical chance of slightly slowing the progression of dementia, they find it easy to rouse vociferous indignation.

With transplants, however, public indignation does not work this way. There may be a certain amount of hand wringing about waiting lists, and the occasional heart-rending story about a particular individual—usually a child—who urgently needs a transplant. But the stories that can be relied on to stir up public anger and anxiety are not about patients who die on the waiting list, let alone the very many who do not even get that far because they are too far down the order of priorities to have any hope of reaching the top. The stories that reach the headlines are nearly all about the sources of organs, and alleged improprieties in their acquisition: mistakes in transplant registers about conditions specified by potential donors, or organs taken without adequate permission, or doubts about whether some donor really was dead. When such things happen the emphasis is entirely on the wrongs alleged to have been done to the sources of the organs or their relatives. There is usually no mention at all of the people whose lives were probably saved by the organs that were said to have been improperly obtained.

This is not surprising. Outrage is a response not just to bad events, but to the feeling that someone is to blame for them. If we think that the state has an obligation to provide everyone with any medical treatment that might benefit them, we can claim that the government could easily provide all the drugs and treatment necessary if only it would (according to political outlook) cut defence spending, impose large taxes on bankers, or thwart welfare cheats. It is easy to demand rights when someone else has the corresponding duty.

But when patients need not just more resources in general, but parts of other people, the matter is different. To provide more organs in a reliable way, governments would have to start encroaching on what the potential sources of these organs regard as their own rights. If the only way a state can guarantee enough organs for transplants is to start depriving us of our rights to keep our bodies out of other people's hands, we are not likely to blame the ever-lengthening waiting lists on government negligence. Of course any of us may need organs at some time, but there seems to be a deep human tendency to be more concerned with holding on to what we have than considering what we might need at some time in the future. Public passion about transplantation is directed towards making sure that all organs are, to use a currently fashionable phrase, ethically sourced.

The organ shortage

Most people are, in principle, all in favour of transplants, at least to the extent that if they have organ failure they will hope for one. But transplants are dependent on organs' being given, and we all know, because we are always being told, that there are nothing like enough of them. Even though a single deceased donor can ideally provide organs to save half a dozen living patients, the donor category is nowhere near large enough to meet the needs of would-be recipients. Many more people could benefit from transplants than have the faintest hope of doing so. Similar claims can be made about all areas of medical treatment, of course, given the ever-expanding demand and the inequitable distribution of medical resources; but even within the constraints of existing medical provision, far more transplants would take place if there were enough available organs.

As a result, what might be called the broad transplant community—the friends and families of the patients deteriorating and dying on waiting lists, the clinicians who could save them if only the means were available, and the former patients who have experienced the transformation a successful transplant can make—are all endlessly considering ways to get more organs. (The patients themselves, it should be said, are usually too ill to campaign on their own behalf.) However, all the enthusiastic advocates of transplantation know they have to tread very carefully, and not seem too rapacious in their organ hunt. They must perpetually reassure a suspicious public that nothing will be done without their consent, and must consider all new possibilities for organ procurement from the point of view of the popular media that constitute the mouthpiece of indignant gut reactions. The slightest hint that any mark has been overstepped in the procurement of organs—any suggestion that they may have been taken without permission or insensitively, or that the need for organs may have affected the treatment of potential donors—might result in a huge backlash and a still greater shortage.

This careful approach means that even the people most committed to transplantation tend not to push for more aggressive procurement policies. Instead they work through task forces and commissions, trying to achieve increased donation rates by instigating schemes to raise public awareness, setting up donation registers, and training transplant coordinators in approaching relatives. It is emphasized over and over again that transplantation depends on a generous gift ('the gift of life'). Nobody has any right to demand your organs, but it would be a noble and altruistic act if you, or your surviving relatives, chose to offer them. The hope is to persuade more and more of the public into the frame of mind that the transplant community is already in, of regarding it as obviously better to recycle the organs of the dead for the benefit of the living than to waste them by burial or burning.

Of course this is all to the good. If individuals can be persuaded to make different choices when the subject of donation comes up, many more lives will be saved. But the choices made by individuals are just the surface of the problem. If people made different choices within the range open to them there would of course be more organs available, but these choices are, like all choices, made against particular social, legal, and institutional backgrounds. People make decisions according to the options open to them, but those options themselves are to a large extent determined by how society is arranged and regulated, and how other people are likely to react.

If we want more organs for transplant, we need to think not just about persuading individuals, but also about the institutional framework against which their choices are made. That is where the fundamental problems of transplant ethics lie, and what this book is about.

Practical ethics

In ordinary life ethics is typically thought of as a top-down enterprise, where you start with a set of moral standards or principles and then apply them to particular situations. The idea is that when you are trying to decide what to do—if you care about ethics—you compare possible courses of action with those standards, and choose the one most in line with them. If you are judging other people you say their actions are ethical or unethical, moral or immoral,* right or wrong, good or bad, by applying your moral standards to them in this way.

In everyday contexts that may indeed be more or less what goes on. We use 'ethical'—or 'moral', or 'right', or 'good'—as a term of approval for whatever meets the standards we are using. But to do this we need to presuppose a particular set of standards; and the question can always be asked of whether those standards are themselves right. This is a question that has always worried philosophers—along with the related problems of whether the question even has any meaning, and how, if at all, it might be answered—but most people, most of the time, have not thought much about it. They have just taken their background standards for granted. Now, however, the deeper questions about which standards to accept have become increasingly hard to avoid in everyday life. This is partly because of the mingling of different cultures with different moral standards, but also partly because science and technology are producing radically new kinds of question to which no traditional standards seem to be able to give clear or satisfactory answers.

There are various kinds of response to these difficulties. One, probably the commonest, is just to reinforce the ramparts around the standards you and your group already hold, forcing new problems into shapes that allow you to make judgements on them, and

---

* I shall be treating 'moral' and 'ethical' as more or less synonymous throughout. There may be slight differences between them in ordinary usage, but none that are consistent enough to be useful here.

using those standards to declare everyone else's competing standards wrong. Another response is to try to embrace some kind of relativism, and claim that everyone's views are 'equally valid' and deserving of equal respect. That one, despite its popularity, cannot even be formulated coherently.[†] A third response is to head for the philosophical stratosphere in search of Ultimate Moral Truth, in the hope that you will at least find out whether there is such a thing, and if so, make some progress in catching it.

This third response may be fine as a matter of intellectual theory; but in the meantime practical people like doctors and politicians must remain in the real world, beset every moment with practical decisions that have to be made immediately. Most philosophers who set off for the stratosphere never return to earth to enlighten the people they have left behind, and the ones who do seem to disagree with each other, so they are not much help. The few practical people who have taken short courses in ethics pick up a smattering of theory that lets them say things like 'if you are Kantian, you do this, if you are a utilitarian you do that...' which, apart from hardly ever being true (because these are types of ethical theory, rather

---

[†] Relativism, as opposed to outright scepticism, is usually expressed in such assertions as 'we should respect everyone's values equally', or 'you shouldn't impose your values on other people'. But:

(1) it is usually very easy to find some value the speaker will refuse to respect—Nazism, for instance.

(2) It is anyway impossible to respect in practice many conflicting values. How could the US President respect equally the values of the anti-abortionists who want to kill abortionists, and pro-abortion campaigners who think that women should not have to bear unwanted children?

(3) The view is anyway self-refuting: the claim that we *should* respect everyone's views equally is itself an expression of an (incoherent) moral view.

than particular moral standards), is of not the slightest use to someone who has no idea whether to be Kantian or a utilitarian, but nevertheless has to decide whether to turn off the ventilator of a potential organ donor, or try to change the donor register to one that works by opting out. So it is not surprising if people with decisions to make regard philosophers as inhabiting a fantasy world of their own, irrelevant to real life.

My own view is that it is hopeless to try to deal with the problems of bioethics—or any other area of practical ethics—in this top-down way. We need to start where everyone else starts, with the practical problems themselves, and then see how much progress can be made make by working from the ground up. That, however, emphatically does not mean ignoring the theoretical problems and just relying on common sense or 'professional judgement'. There are things to be learned about the analysis of ethical problems, and discoveries to be made about moral reasoning, that can have as much effect on the way we think and act as do the scientific discoveries that confront us with the problems.

What this book attempts to do is propose and demonstrate a method for doing some of these things. It is intended primarily not as a defence of a particular set of views but as a way of working through the problems, and it should in theory work equally well for everyone. It is unlikely to produce agreement, but it should at least make clear where the roots of disagreement lie, and the nature of the problems that need to be resolved.

There is no point in trying to explain many of the details of this method in abstract; it will be better to plunge directly into the problems themselves, and consider afterwards how the arguments have worked. Still, it may be useful to start with a brief introduction to the approach.

The method of enquiry

One of the great problems about discussions of practical ethics, which are often full of passion, is keeping the arguments in order. Practical problems are usually presented—in conferences, for instance, and in the media—as pro-and-con debates in which people take sides about matters of policy. This is supposed to provide balance, and present 'both sides of the argument', but what usually results is what Winnie the Pooh might describe as a Confused Noise. Incompatible arguments get heaped up on each side as though they reinforced each other, replies to opponents mix up objections to the conclusion with objections to particular arguments in defence of the conclusion, and both sides slither between arguments about the problem itself and speculations about the other side's motives. The issues get lost in the psychology of warfare.

It may be inevitable that practical politics falls into this form, given the kind of creature we are, but anyone who is morally serious needs to work out what is worth achieving before going into the politics of trying to achieve it. The ethical enquiry that should precede practical politics must concentrate on the problems themselves, not the matter of sides, and that means getting the issues into a format that is above all concerned with clarity. If people come to different practical conclusions, we need to know where in the background the roots of their disagreements lie. If we are puzzled as individuals about what practical conclusion to reach, we need to know what kind of enquiry would help to resolve the problem.

There is no single way of going about this kind of clarification, and it is extraordinarily difficult to do in the linear format necessary for a book. You know that anything you say about a difficult subject will be met by a chorus of 'Oh but...'s, as readers think of swarms of different objections to what they think you have said. Even though you may have anticipated all their points, and will gradually get to them, you can deal with only one at a time—and in the process you may lose the people who have thought of other 'Oh but...'s, and concluded that since you have missed their obvious point there is not much purpose in going on. The only satisfactory way I have found of conducting a complex and contentious practical argument in public is to have an enormous blackboard, the whole width of a lecture theatre (white boards, flip charts, and PowerPoint are absolutely no substitute), and write on it everything everyone says. Then no one can think their point has been lost, and you can later draw lines showing how the various elements of argument connect together, and where the problems come. In a book, you can only hope that the reader will persevere.

What I propose to do here is put the analysis into a format that I think will allow for everything anyone will want to say, even if the starting point and method are unfamiliar. This should cast the problems in a different light, and in doing so, I hope, demonstrate how moral reasoning—from the ground up, not the top down—can make real progress.

I shall take as a starting proposition the claim that if someone's life or health can be saved by means of a transplant, that is in itself a good thing.

That needs immediate clarification. I am not suggesting that if you need a transplant, and I could give you one by murdering someone and passing their organs on to you, that is what I should do. There is an important distinction between something's being good or bad *in one way* and its being good or bad *all things considered*. Even the murder would be good in one way if your life were saved. There would be something good about what happened—one good aspect to the overall situation—even though not many people would say that the situation was good *all things considered*, or that I had done the right thing in murdering someone else to save you. In saying that it is a good thing to save someone's life by a transplant I mean only that it is *intrinsically* good, or good *in itself*: that whatever else is true of the situation overall, that aspect of it is good. It is intrinsically good to save your life.

When the claim is understood in this way, it should be clear that it is absolutely minimal. It involves no claim about *how* good or important saving a life is in comparison with other things—just that it is generally good in itself. I suppose it is theoretically possible that some people might not accept even this, and be against the whole principle of saving lives and alleviating suffering by means of transplants, though I have never actually come across any. If so, however, there is no point in their reading this book—and I doubt whether they would have bothered to look at it in the first place. Everyone actually involved in debates about transplantation takes the *intrinsic* value of saving lives and restoring health, and therefore of doing this by transplantation, as given.

It follows from this that if someone is dying or ill, and could be saved for a life worth living by a transplant, there is a *presumption* in favour of bringing that about whenever possible. If we add to that the fact that there is a severe shortage of organs, and many people die who could be saved if more were available, that generates a presumption in favour of any policy that opens up a potential source of organs, and conversely against any policy that closes or curtails one.

This also needs immediate clarification. A presumption is only that: it is potentially defeasible. If you knew nothing more about some practice than that it involved sticking needles into children, your presumption, pending further evidence, would be that it should be stopped. You would probably withdraw your objection when you saw that nothing more sinister was going on than vaccination or the administration of anaesthesia, whose benefits far outweighed the intrinsic harm—but you would want the evidence first. Similarly, the claim that there is a presumption in favour of any means of getting organs for transplant does not begin to suggest that we should go ahead with them all. It implies only that if we accept that it is good in itself to save people by transplants, the *burden of proof* lies on anyone who wants to block or impede some particular means of getting organs. They need to show that *even though people will suffer and die* as a result of that obstruction, it is nevertheless justified.

Setting the matter up in this way makes no difference to the substance of the debate. There may well be a good justification for blocking some particular means of procurement, and if there is such a justification it will appear. But the approach is methodologically useful, just because—as already suggested—people are much more likely to complain about methods of procuring organs than about lives lost and illness suffered as a result of their unavailability. If we have such general tendencies, it is useful to have a methodology that subjects these natural inclinations to proper scrutiny by starting with a presumption in favour of getting organs whenever we can.

That raises the question of whether the presumption can be defeated; and in some contexts a decisive objection comes so immediately that it is easy to overlook the fact that the presumption even exists. If I suggest murdering someone to get their organs, you will probably rule the idea out so quickly that it will simply not occur to you that there might have been anything at all to be said in its favour. But what that actually amounts to, in this context, is giving no thought to the people who will suffer and die as a result of not getting those organs, and they deserve at least recognition. Being aware that justification is needed for policies that result in suffering and death is an important starting point. If you recognize it explicitly, you also see the need to make your objections explicit, and check whether they really do justify the resulting harm to potential recipients.

I doubt whether many people would want to challenge the objection to murder even if they thought about it with great care; but in other cases supposedly overriding objections may be presented just as quickly but be much more open to question. It is therefore useful to look at all cases from this point of view, and consider carefully any obstructions and impediments to organ procurement. Even if doing this does not make us change our minds about what is and is not acceptable, it will at least force us to think things through; and when the world changes as radically as it has done in making body parts transferable between people, radical thinking is needed.

Here are two opening illustrations of how the process works.

The first is a variation on a proposal made by John Harris some years ago.[1] Harris pointed out that since any of us might need a transplant at some time in our lives, we could all increase our statistical life expectancy by agreeing to be registered for what he called a *Survival Lottery*. Whenever half a dozen people needing transplants could be saved by the organs of a single person, lots would be drawn to see which healthy individual should be sacrificed to save the six in need. The chances of anyone's being drawn in the lottery would be far lower than that of their dying prematurely of organ failure at some point in their lives. Interestingly, however, it seems that nobody confronted with this thought experiment would choose to join any such scheme.

Imagine this as a proposal not for an optional arrangement, but for an official state policy, with everyone compulsorily enrolled. If you start with the presumption in favour of saving lives by getting more transplant organs, you get an argument on these lines:

> It is intrinsically good to save lives.
>
> If we had enough organs, transplantation could save many more lives than it currently does.
>
> We could save all these lives, and increase everyone's statistical life expectancy, if we instituted some kind of survival lottery.
>
> --------------------
>
> Therefore (presumptively) we should institute a survival lottery.

Everyone, presumably, would accept the argument's premises. The first is a value claim, about what matters, which I am treating— when properly understood—as uncontroversial. The second two are claims about empirical facts—about what the world is like and how it works—and they are both true. However nobody, it seems, would accept the conclusion these premises seem to support. So how can we avoid accepting it?

When the problem is presented in this form, it is clear that what is needed is an added 'But…' premise, that would defeat the presumption and support the opposite conclusion. Given that most of us would be horrified at the idea of implementing the conclusion, while the premises seem so innocuous, it is at least interesting to see what kind of premise we might insert to justify the opposite conclusion.

So the challenge is to find an argument of this form:

It is intrinsically good to save lives.

If we had enough organs, transplantation could save many more lives than it currently does.

We could save all these lives, and increase everyone's statistical life expectancy, if we instituted some kind of survival lottery.

But…

Therefore we should *not* institute a survival lottery.

We need to find some way of filling the 'But…' premise that is both acceptable in itself and does the logical job of overriding the presumption and supporting the conclusion. Until that is done, the presumption in favour of a survival lottery remains undefeated.

So, if you are against the idea of a survival lottery, how would you complete the argument? My own response, for what it is worth, would break down into two elements: a factual claim about human nature, and a moral claim about the significance of the factual claim.

The factual claim is that it seems to be simply a truth about human nature that there are many things we care about a great deal more than life expectancy. We know this from everyday experience—or we would never go rock climbing, or drive, or smoke, or eat fatty foods—but some of the things we turn out to care about are interestingly unexpected. A real proposal, similar in some ways to the survival lottery, was made in the Second World War,[2] in a context where a pilot's chance of surviving thirty high-risk bombing missions was only one in four. 'It was calculated that one-way missions, by reducing the fuel load, could increase the load of bombs, so that only half the pilots need fly. Selection would be by lot, with half the pilots escaping altogether and the other half going to certain death.' The arrangement would double each pilot's chance of surviving the war; but still the plan was not put into practice, and this will probably surprise nobody. Most people would probably prefer to keep to the original arrangement if they were in that position, in spite of the much higher chance of mortality, and it is interesting to consider why. Perhaps we would want to keep hope going until the last moment; perhaps as individuals we would feel that we could do better if our fate remained in our own hands. But whatever the reason, it seems to be a simple fact about most people that our strong preferences would take that form, and would survive any amount of consideration.

Our reaction to the Survival Lottery is striking in similar ways. It may surprise us to discover that we prefer a greater chance of a slow and unpleasant death by organ failure than a much lower probability of death—which could be quick, painless, and even unannounced—by losing a lottery, and the discovery is an interesting contribution to our ever-expanding understanding of human nature. But still, if our concern is to make arrangements that suit our species as it actually is, not some other species whose overriding values are different, extending life expectancy does not provide a justification for imposing a survival lottery. So I would be inclined to complete the argument along these lines:

It is intrinsically good to save lives.

If we had enough organs, transplantation could save many more lives than it currently does.

We could save all these lives, and increase everyone's statistical life expectancy, if we instituted some kind of survival lottery.

But...   *It seems to be a deep fact about human nature that we regard many things as more important than life expectancy, and, even with full understanding and after careful consideration, few people would be willing to purchase additional life expectancy at the cost of entering a survival lottery.*

We should not put in place arrangements that would please nobody.

Therefore we should *not* institute a survival lottery.

The first added premise is a claim about the facts of the matter: a claim about the deep preferences people (at least currently) seem to have. The second is a value claim, which, if you accept it, overrides the presumption that we should maximize the saving of lives. The two together defeat the initial presupposition that there should be a survival lottery.

Of course even this does not mean the argument has reached an end. You might challenge either of the proposed added premises. You might claim that this was not a deep fact about human nature, and that once we got used to the idea we would be perfectly happy. You might claim that fulfilling people's deep preferences was not the right moral value, and that some other value was better. Or you might add other considerations. Perhaps if we had just had a catastrophic nuclear war or been hit by a meteorite, and the human race was in danger of dying out, you might decide that nothing was more important than life expectancy and that people's personal feelings must be overridden. But at least getting the problem into this form would show where the scope for doubt and disagreement lay. A puzzled individual, thinking through the problem, would know what kind of work was needed to resolve it; people who disagreed about the conclusion would see where in the background the roots of their disagreement lay. This approach at least gets the matter clear, and that is the beginning of any rational enquiry.

Anyway, quite irrespective of where you think the debate should go from there, it is an interesting challenge to explain why the argument for the survival lottery does not work, rather than just rejecting it because it feels wrong. That is what this book is about. Many people have strong feelings about controversial issues in the transplant debate, and this way of going about things presents a challenge to them to articulate exactly what their position is.

Here is another illustration, which may be more puzzling. When I first became involved in these issues, I found at one international transplant meeting that great horror was being expressed about the regular use in China of organs from executed criminals. More recently China has claimed that this no longer happens, but people suspect it does, and the idea is still widely regarded as outrageous. Whatever the truth, the ethics of the matter is worth consideration.

Of course if you are against capital punishment altogether you will regard the whole business as terrible: you will see it as akin to murdering people for their organs. (Murder is, after all, illicit killing, so what counts as murder is determined by the ethical system that says whether or not something should be treated as illicit.) If you have no objection to capital punishment as such, but suspect that it is used too often in China for the specific purpose of increasing organ procurement, you will also think many of the executions are wrong. But in either of those cases your objection is to the unjustified executions themselves, not to the subsequent use of the organs; and what was striking about the protests was that the people involved did not seem to be complaining about the executions themselves. They were apparently concerned to stop the transplants irrespective of whether the executions went on. The interesting question here, therefore, is not about the all-things-considered justifiability of what was happening in China (about which we may not know enough), but about whether there is an objection to using the organs of executed prisoners *even if* (or perhaps irrespective of whether) the executions are justified.

Suppose the Chinese defended their practice like this:

There is a presumption in favour of getting more organs for transplant.

One way to do this is to use of the organs of executed prisoners.

Therefore we should use the organs of executed prisoners.

What '*But…*' premise could be inserted in that argument, to reverse the conclusion?

What was being said at the time was that the prisoners had not given valid consent—and, indeed, since they were prisoners, that they *could not* give valid consent. So the implied argument seemed to be something like this:

There is a presumption in favour of getting more organs for transplant.

One way to do that is to make use of the organs of executed prisoners.

But…   *Valid consent is an absolute requirement for the use of organs.*

These people have not given, and because they are prisoners cannot give, valid consent.

Therefore we should *not* use the organs of executed prisoners.

The matter of valid consent will come up later, but for the moment assume that the prisoners in question were not even asked, and gave no consent of any kind, so that the second added premise is true. What, then, about the first? It is a moral claim, but is it obviously one that should be accepted? We may accept that we should normally have the right not to have our organs used even after death unless we consent (though that itself is controversial); but of course we also normally have the right not to be killed. Prisoners do not usually consent to being executed. If it is legitimate for the state to deprive people of life irrespective of their consent, what is the basis of a claim that it is obviously wrong to deprive them (posthumously) of their organs without their consent? Most people would regard that as a far less important right than the right to life. If you think that people can deserve to die for their crimes, why should they not deserve to lose their organs as well—thereby, indeed, returning some good to society, by saving other lives?

Perhaps the response to this might be that there was nothing in Chinese law to allow for this removal of organs without consent. But the Chinese might argue that the use of organs was an implicit part of a death sentence. Or, if not, that it could be added as part of the sentence—in the way that British criminals in the eighteenth century could be sentenced to dissection as well as execution. Would that make it acceptable? If not, what is the moral basis of a claim that execution can be an appropriate punishment, but that organ retrieval without consent cannot be? What if the Chinese added to their list of punishments compulsory organ retrieval after death, but without any hastening of death? It would be quite extraordinary if there were international protests about punishment by compulsory use of organs after natural death, but not about punishment by killing.

This kind of analysis, when there is a passionate and strong reaction to some organ-getting policy, is usually illuminating. In this case, if you have such a response, the approach starts by getting you to clarify exactly what your complaint is: execution, or execution to get organs, or just taking organs without consent. Even to work out your own position you need to recognize these as distinct issues. And then, even if you feel strongly that execution can be justified, but that taking organs without consent cannot be, it at least gets you to confront the question of how you could justify such an odd principle about what really mattered, and which human rights should be treated as absolutely inalienable. Furthermore, putting the whole problem into an argument of this form—with a presumption in favour of saving lives by getting organs—shows that you need to explain not only why you think posthumous organ requisition should be regarded as a more serious violation of human rights than execution, but also why respecting this right as absolute is more important than saving the lives of half a dozen innocent, sick people by means of transplants.

As someone who is against execution altogether, I personally think that if people are to be executed it is better that their organs should be used than wasted, and that the Chinese might reasonably accuse places like the United States of wantonly sacrificing, or at least failing to save, the lives of innocent, sick citizens by not using the organs of the people it regards as deserving execution. But it would be clear where I and anyone who thought otherwise disagreed. Spelling out the arguments like this does help to clarify difficulties and disagreements by pulling them out of the fog of uncritical emotion.

This also suggests why going through arguments in this way may not lead everyone to the same conclusion: there may turn out to be moral disagreements at a deeper level. But it also forces the examination of moral assumptions in ways that can lead to mind changing. I would like to think that by the end of the book such arguments and analyses will have led some people to change their minds in unexpected ways, and also that some apparent disagreements may not be as deep as they seem.

Assorted caveats

Finally, I should make clear what the book does *not* attempt to do. It is an extended analytical essay whose aim is to shift the way matters of transplantation are discussed and thought about, and many topics that might be dealt with by a book on transplants are not covered here.

First, the book is not a source of facts about transplantation, either clinical or organizational. It does not go into any of the physiological details, or the practical arrangements and problems, or statistics about waiting lists and life expectancy after transplantation. Nor does it attempt to discuss the legal background in different countries, or to describe the extent of differences of social backgrounds, or moral standards, or cultural attitudes to transplantation. I shall attempt to explain in which contexts factual information of certain sorts is relevant, but not to give that information. I shall refer to illustrations of laws and attitudes and institutional arrangements, but only in the sketchiest of terms for the purpose of analysing them, not with any intention of making claims about how widespread any of them is, or how much they vary. The illustrations tend to be UK-centric, as those are the ones with which I am most familiar but even those do not attempt any accuracy of detail. The purpose is to discuss debates about types of policy, not to describe actual policies.

Second, my concern here is specifically with the *procurement* of organs for transplant—not the innumerable other moral issues that come up in the context of transplantation. In particular, I shall say very little about the question of allocation—who should receive the organs that are available—even though this question has enormous practical importance. I shall also say nothing at all about such general matters as the treatment of children and mentally incompetent patients, or address wider questions about the use of resources, because these are questions that arise in all areas of medicine in broadly similar ways. Here I concentrate on what I take to be the distinctive problem of transplantation: that of organ procurement. There are comparable issues in the context of fertility treatments, of course, with sperm and egg donation and surrogacy, but those are sufficiently different to need separate treatment. Another issue I shall not deal with, mainly because of limited space, is the procurement and use of tissues such as skin and cells of various kinds, as opposed to whole organs intended to perform their original function in a new body. The issues are closely related, since tissues as well as organs must have sources, but the difference between the two subjects seems great enough to call for their being treated separately.‡

Third, the book is a work of practical ethics, dependent on philosophical techniques in the analysis of argument, but it makes no attempt to provide an overview of the bioethical literature in this area, or to engage with it. There is a huge amount of this literature now, generated partly by the medical profession and partly by philosophers, but I do not go into it at all. The structure and

---

‡ Having worked through the arguments of Ch. 4, I now suspect that the relevant distinction may be between use for treatment and use for research rather than between organs and tissues, but that will take more investigation.

content of the book are rooted entirely in its origins in popular and medical debate, in broadcasts, blogs, and medical (as opposed to philosophical) conferences. The way the arguments are developed here arises entirely from interactions and discussions in these contexts, and often ideas and claims discussed will not be attributed or even attributable. That will not matter, however, because the point is not to describe the state of public or professional opinion (which is, of course, extremely variable), but to consider the question of what the response should be *if* someone says this or that. All the ideas discussed are in the air at the moment, but it is not relevant to my purpose to make any claims how prevalent any of them are. I have deliberately kept references to an absolute minimum, so that the discussion is fixed on the issues themselves rather than any particular expression of them.

One consequence of this approach is that the book presupposes no knowledge of philosophical ethics. The fundamental techniques of philosophy are just developments of ordinary reasoning, and nothing beyond that appears here. Anyone can follow these arguments. All that is needed is a serious engagement with the issues, and a willingness to penetrate the impressionistic fog of argument that develops when people are bent on defending, rather than testing, their moral intuitions. It will not be of much interest to anyone looking only for confirmation of what they already believe.

It is perhaps also worth commenting on the language and tone of the book, since I have many times found that unfamiliarity of language and purpose causes serious misunderstanding across the huge (highly regrettable) cultural gulf between medicine and practical philosophy. Because this book is intended as a pre-political enquiry—intended to clarify what is worth fighting about before the fighting starts—it is important to avoid any of the tendentious language that is rhetorically useful for the purpose of persuasion, but which seriously distorts enquiry. For that reason, I shall on the whole avoid using 'donor' and 'donation' as general terms, because if we are considering how to get organs we should not start by presupposing that all acceptable acquisition must involve a gift. Perhaps donation may be the only acceptable method of procurement, but that is one of the questions at issue. We need neutral terms, such as 'source' for the person the organs come from, and 'procurement' for the business of getting them—with donation as just one possible method of procurement, and donors as just one possible source. Similarly, there is no simple alternative for the rather stark 'cadaveric' to describe organs taken from the dead. The gentler 'deceased' is fine for referring to the sources of the organs, but 'deceased kidney' sounds rather odd. Language must no doubt be adapted to the purposes of political persuasion when that stage is reached, but here the arguments are addressed only to people who are trying to decide what political ends should be pursued.

Perhaps it should also be remarked—about a different matter of language—that the nearest I have found to a satisfactory sex-neutral pronoun is treating 'they' as singular. The politically correct alternation of 'he' and 'she', now widely adopted by philosophers, seems to me intolerably clumsy. The singular use of 'they' could, I think, become acceptable (we have a precedent in 'you', which used to be only plural), and although it is still too awkward to use in many places, there are some contexts where it seems to work. Jane Austen does it, and that is good enough for me.

Jane Austen also brings to mind another thought. Given all the caveats about what this book will *not* be doing, it may sound as though it will also amount to working with a fine brush on a two-inch piece of ivory, and as such too limited to be of much significance. I hope to show that this is not the case, and that such a modest enterprise can have surprising results. At least, several of them have surprised me.

2

PROCUREMENT FROM THE LIVING

Established rights

The most obvious laws that prevent our getting enough organs for transplant—so obvious that it does not occur to us to think of them in that way—are the ones that place a circle of rights round living individuals to prevent inappropriate encroachment by others. There are, after all, plenty of organs around—we are all full of them—but long before transplantation became a possibility there were laws in place that automatically had the effect of protecting us from anyone who might later be tempted to think of us as repositories of transplantable organs. Laws against murder have been around for ever, and if you are protected against murder you are *ipso facto* protected against being murdered for your organs. There are also equally ancient rules of various sorts against what might be loosely described as invading other people's protected space or limiting their freedom without their consent; and if you are protected against bodily invasion or false imprisonment, those laws as they stand protect you from being kidnapped for the forcible removal of a kidney. Transplantation came into a world already full of obstructions to getting organs from living people.

If the moral questions are really to be explored from the foundations, then, the advent of transplantation suggests we should reconsider these laws. The essence of rights is that they override, or trump, considerations that would otherwise be regarded as important. If you have the right to keep people out of your house, that trumps their need for shelter; if people accused of crimes have the right to be regarded as innocent until proved guilty, that trumps the preference the rest of us might have for pre-emptive incarceration of suspicious characters. All rights have costs, and when we are deciding what rights people should have, we need to judge whether they are worth those costs. This is why, although people always want rights for themselves, they are much less sure about universal rights. Although your rights benefit you, the fact that other people have them as well imposes costs on you.

So, if we are to take the enquiry systematically, and recognize a presumption against any policy that restricts the availability of transplant organs, we should start by acknowledging that there are costs to our being protected against being killed or captured for our organs. As the idea of the Survival Lottery shows, we could all increase our statistical life expectancy if we allowed the killing of one individual whenever we needed a set of organs that could save several others. The law is already familiar with the idea of defences that make some cases of deliberate killing not count as murder, so the presumption in favour of organ procurement might suggest that we should consider extending such a defence to surgeons who sent out hit squads whenever they accumulated half a dozen patients who could be saved by the organs of a single victim. We could even build in a specification that the defence should apply only in cases where the victim was caught and killed so quickly and unexpectedly that there would be no fear or suffering.

But, as I have said, most people, however much they thought about the probabilities, would find they would rather keep the absolute protection against deliberate killing that we have now. However mysterious it may be, if we would all prefer to have a higher probability of dying slowly and unpleasantly of natural causes than a significantly lower probability of being killed painlessly and instantaneously for our organs, that seems to settle the matter.

Perhaps, then, there might be more plausible scope for wondering about the legal protection we now have against lesser encroachments than killing. Very early in the history of successful transplantation it was discovered that some organs could be taken from living donors with only the slightest chance of killing them or even doing them lasting harm. Kidney donation, in particular, involves an operation that is only minimally risky in itself, and with proper follow-up does no long-term harm because the remaining kidney expands to take over the function of the other. This presents rather more interesting possibilities. Perhaps there might be a lesser version of the survival lottery that did not involve killing. We might alter the law so that whenever anyone needed a kidney, some random person was drawn in a lottery to be the donor. This would not involve killing anyone—only some temporary pain and inconvenience, for which, let us say for the sake of argument, the victim could be amply compensated. That would raise everyone's statistical life expectancy, and involve no deaths or long-term harm at all. Might we then reduce the protection we currently have against assault and battery, to allow for this?

This is a much more modest proposal, and I can imagine that some people might be interested in setting up an optional version of such an arrangement—although under present law it would probably come into the category of unenforceable contract, as in the case of arrangements that are made for the bearing of children by surrogate mothers. However, as long as such an arrangement was voluntary it would still keep the consent requirement intact, and that is the essence of the matter here. My guess is that if there were any question of removing or lessening the protective circle of rights that prevents other people from making unauthorized inroads into our bodies, even with such a minimal probability of its actually happening and considerable compensation if it did, most people would respond nearly as negatively as to the idea of the full-blown Survival Lottery. If so, this once again throws an interesting light on human nature: an illumination of social structures that we regard as more valuable than extended life expectancy, and whose desirability, for most of us, survives even long reflection. It does seem that the wish for protection of bodily integrity against other people is something that most people regard as fundamental, as with the protection from being killed. If so, once again, that seems to me to settle the matter.

Anyway, these fundamental rights are not among the obstructions to organ procurement that I want to challenge here—which is no doubt just as well, since bioethicists look more and more irrelevant if their recommendations move too far away from what people want for themselves. These entrenched obstructions to procurement, which consist of rights to protection that everyone has and seems to want, are mentioned only for the sake of completeness, and for contrast with other kinds of obstruction.

The really interesting questions about restrictions on organ procurement from the living are of the opposite kind. They concern the various contexts in which people *are* willing to consent to organ donation, but are still not allowed to do it.

Established restrictions

The first set of restrictions that comes into this category is, like the laws against murder and assault, one that was in place long before there was any possibility of transplantation, but which also has the effect of limiting some possibilities for organ procurement. These are the laws that limit the amount of harm one person may do to another, even though that other may be willing, or even eager, to offer consent.

It is useful here to distinguish between formal, legal constraints and the ones that reflect the policies and decisions of individual practitioners. All reputable transplant centres screen prospective living donors with some care, and many possible donors are rejected in consequence. Many centres, for instance, have a long-standing suspicion of so-called Samaritan (or, increasingly, 'altruistic') donors: people who appear out of nowhere and offer a kidney for a stranger in need. For all the emphasis on altruism and generosity in the field of organ donation, there seems also to be a feeling that anyone who wants to offer a kidney in this way must be unbalanced or have ulterior motives, and this leads to the refusal of many donations that are offered. In other cases the clinical team may regard the risks to the health of the donor as greater than it is willing to allow, in spite of the donor's understanding of the situation and wish to proceed nevertheless. The doctors involved may also be worried about the circumstances of particular cases: afraid, perhaps, that the donor may be planning to exploit the recipient later, or has been misled by an appearance of friendship and attachment that might disappear once the donation had been made.

These cases are all interesting, and, given the starting presumption in favour of organ procurement, all raise questions about the justifiability of the decisions. We may have doubts about the medical paternalism involved; we may think people should have the right to give a kidney if they want to. But for now, at least, doctors are in most circumstances entitled to decide whether or not they perform a particular procedure. A surgeon cannot operate without the patient's consent, but, equally, the patient needs an offer to consent to. Whatever their reasons, the transplant team can veto any offered donation. It would involve a considerable change to try to force doctors to do what, as individual professionals, they were unwilling to do.

However, that still leaves the more fundamental problem of cases where a patient is willing to consent to some procedure, and the surgeon is also willing to go ahead, but the law nevertheless will not allow it. There are laws that prevent one person from harming (maiming) or killing another, even with that person's consent and by their desire. These laws are general, like the laws against murder and battery, but like them they automatically have the effect of restricting some possible cases of living organ retrieval. In fact they seemed at first to rule out even the kinds of living kidney and liver donation that are now routine, since, on the face of it, removal of a kidney or liver lobe for non-therapeutic purposes constituted grievous bodily harm; but it seems to have been tacitly accepted everywhere that the minimal risk to the donor, and the enormous benefit to the recipient, makes transplantation an acceptable defence for such infliction of harm. But it is still not clear how far the law will stretch, and transplant teams—quite apart from any of their own concerns about inflicting harm on patients—are naturally cautious about the law. Surgeons refused, for instance, to take the second kidney of a father who had already made a donation to one son, and now wanted to give his other kidney to a second son whose kidney had failed, even though the father would not die but take his son's place on dialysis.[1] And the law would certainly not allow the removal of any organ, such as a heart, that was essential for the life of the donor. 'A man may declare himself ready to die for another, but the surgeon must not take him at his word.'[2]

These issues are of considerable theoretical interest. There is no mystery about the fact that there are contexts in which consent is regarded as necessary but not sufficient for some procedure, because in many cases there are clearly implications for other people as well as the person whose consent is necessary. Even though your rights over your own house mean that your consent is needed for (nearly) everything that is done to it or in it, they do not extend to replacing timber window frames with plastic ones in a historic building, or allowing your friend to use your living room for dealing in drugs. Some activities are regarded as of too great interest to others to leave entirely to your own control. And, interestingly, the laws against killing and maiming even with consent were originally seen in more or less this way: offences not primarily against the consenting individual, but against other interested parties. Killing was an offence against God and also the sovereign—suicide was regarded as self-murder—and maiming an offence because it deprived the sovereign of an able-bodied man. (The greatest temptation to consent to harm to yourself was escape from military service.) And because of these other interests, these things were equally offences whether someone else did them to you with your consent or you did them to yourself.

However, even when the underpinning ideas shifted, and laws about what you could legally do to yourself were gradually modified to recognize that the interests involved were primarily your own, the restrictions on what other people could do to you remained. So, for instance, when the 1961 Suicide Act was passed in the UK, suicide and attempted suicide ceased to be criminal offences and were to that extent moved out of the area of public interest and returned to the circle of individual control. But the same Act explicitly stated that 'aiding, abetting, counselling or procuring' the suicide of another remained criminal offences. It also left untouched the classification of euthanasia as murder, even when the person killed had consented to, or even pleaded for, death.

Similarly, self-harm is not generally regarded as a criminal offence, and to that extent the law regards individuals' treatment of themselves as a matter for personal decision. But there are still limits to the amount of harm others can legally do to you, even with your consent. This shows in rulings about harm caused during consensual sado-masochistic activity,[3] and in the uncertain legal situation of surgeons who operate on patients seeking the amputation of normal but unwanted limbs. And since you cannot remove your own organs for transplantation, such restrictions potentially rule out several kinds of organ donation. For instance, in countries that forbid euthanasia and the assisting of suicide, you cannot plan to commit suicide in ways that would reliably make your organs available to other people, because that would require the aiding and abetting of your suicide by the transplant team.

Many people object strongly to restrictions of this kind, regarding them as anomalous hangovers from a pre-Enlightenment past, and inconsistent with present-day ideals of autonomy and liberty. From this point of view, valid consent should be a sufficient condition for allowing others to do what we would like to do to ourselves but cannot, and laws preventing this are just self-indulgence on the part of a nanny state, hanging on to the old rules even though the old justifications have gone. Other people—presumably most governments—think there is sufficient justification in spite of the change in underpinning justification (which, of course, they may not even have noticed).

Such restrictions may have relatively little effect on the availability of organs for transplant, but they certainly block some possibilities. Pressure for change in legislation against euthanasia and assisting suicide is increasing all the time, and it seems likely that many of the people who press for these rights would want them to include the option of linking them with organ donation. In countries that allow euthanasia, such as Belgium, organs are already being retrieved for transplant, by the patients' own desire. If you decide to commit suicide, which is not illegal, it is at least on the face of it absurd that you should not be able to do it in a way that saves half a dozen other lives. There are also other possibilities. Many parents, for instance, are willing to make enormous sacrifices for their children and might even be willing to die for them.

However, I shall not go further into this question here, because the laws in question are general, with a scope extending far beyond transplantation, and probably only marginally significant for the matter of procurement. They are mentioned here—like the laws that protect the living from encroachment and murder—mainly for the sake of completeness, and for the sake of contrast with the next set of obstructions to transplantation. These are much more interesting from the point of view of organ procurement, and in some cases highly significant.

New restrictions

This third set of obstructions to organ procurement consists of ones that are not incidental implications of pre-existing laws, but were introduced specially to prevent kinds of organ procurement that would not otherwise have been illegal.

Restrictions that come into this category vary a good deal from country to country. In some places, for instance, living donation is allowed only from relatives. In most places there is a general resistance to allowing organ donation by prisoners. Sometimes there may be specific extra hoops that some categories of potential donors must go through, such as when the UK had its Unrelated Living Transplant Regulatory Authority (ULTRA, now defunct) which required special vetting of any unrelated donor volunteers.[4] Even though this did not rule out unrelated donation, the hoops certainly acted as deterrents to many possible donors and clinicians.

All such restrictions are worth discussion. However, having mentioned the wider category, I shall concentrate on the one that is overwhelmingly the most important in terms of numbers and active concern. This is the widespread, almost universal, prohibition of payment for living kidney donation.

The analysis of this issue will take most of the rest of the chapter. Going through the stages of debate in some detail is the best way both to show how the method of argument outlined in the previous chapter actually works in practice, and, I hope, to demonstrate how moral reasoning can make real progress.

The payment issue

When evidence of the trade in transplant organs from live vendors first filtered through to Western attention some years ago, the most remarkable aspects of the response were its immediacy and apparent unanimity. In the UK this happened in 1989, when it was revealed that two Turkish peasants had come to Harley Street—the London abode of expensive doctors with correspondingly affluent patients—to sell kidneys for patients in need of transplants. Immediately, from all points of the political compass—from widely different groups who were normally hard pressed to agree about anything—there came indignant denunciations of the whole business. It was a moral outrage: a gross exploitation of the poor by the greedy rich, who were now taking the very bodies of those from whom there was nothing else left to take.

There had been no law against such transactions at the time, but the exchange was immediately halted, one of the doctors concerned was struck off the medical register and the other two disciplined, and legislation to ensure that such things never happened again rushed through the UK Parliament with almost unprecedented speed. Professional bodies rapidly declared their anathemas, and soon payment for kidney donation was illegal in most of the world. And because payment for organs has nevertheless continued—legally in a few places, illegally in most—energetic denunciations of it and campaigns against it have continued. The World Health Organization's *Guiding Principles on Human Cell, Tissue and Organ Transplantation* include the principle that 'purchasing, or offering to purchase, cells, tissues or organs for transplantation, or their sale by living persons or by the next of kin for deceased persons, should be banned'.[5] More recently, the *Declaration of Istanbul on Organ Trafficking and Transplant Tourism*[6] also pronounces against allowing payment.

In view of all this, it is interesting to start by considering the matter from the other direction: that of the people who had been engaging in exchange of organs for payment when it first came to light, before it was so widely made illegal.

Transplantation is, seen against the history of our species, a radically new phenomenon. Many body parts, whose only value had been as functioning elements of the person they belonged to, had suddenly changed their status. They could now be transferred to become functioning parts of other people. Most could not be used in this way until the death of the original owner, but a few could even be removed from a living person for transfer to someone else without much risk to the source. And inevitably, as people became aware of these possibilities, they started to recognize new opportunities. Now that organs could be moved between people, in much the same way as other possessions, people would naturally start to think about them in similar ways.

Of course the people who were interested in the new possibilities would include the criminally inclined who might turn their minds to abduction and murder and trafficking—all of which were ruled out by existing laws and decent moral standards quite irrespective of any special concerns with body parts. But, just as naturally, the possibility of ordinary trade, quite legitimate by all normal standards, would also be recognized. If one group of people finds that it is in desperate need of something in short supply, and another group realizes it is in a position to supply that need in a way that can be turned to its own advantage, the two will inevitably recognize the possibilities for mutually beneficial exchange. It is equally natural that yet others should recognize the scope for facilitating such exchanges. A trade was pretty well bound to develop.

Furthermore, no one involved would have had the slightest reason to think there could be any objection. It had already been established as acceptable for a surgeon to remove a kidney for the purpose of transplantation without being prosecuted for committing grievous bodily harm. It also seemed that an organ must be regarded as effectively belonging to its source, since donor consent was both necessary and sufficient to allow the surgeon to go ahead. What is ours to give is also normally ours to sell. There had also been no historical objection to the idea that you were entitled to sell such transferable bodily elements as hair, or breast milk, or even teeth (arguably a much more horrible business, when it happened, than nephrectomy now). So there was absolutely nothing in existing law or convention to suggest that payment for organ donation was not allowable. On the contrary, its permissibility seemed a perfectly reasonable inference from the rules in all other contexts, now that some body parts had changed their status to become more like other kinds of transferable goods.

This prima facie acceptability is also suggested by the very fact that specific laws and policies banning payment for organs had to be introduced at all. When suicide was decriminalized in the UK special laws against assisting suicide had to be added to the Act, because our normal standards would have suggested that if some action was not in itself criminal, neither would be aiding and abetting it. Similarly, because the legal and conventional background provided no general basis whatever for preventing competent adults from making mutually beneficial exchanges, something deliberate had to be done if such exchanges were to be prevented in this particular context.

It is not surprising, then, that payment for organs developed spontaneously, and that the people involved had no reason to think there could be any objection to it. In the light of that, the question arises of what objections can be offered to allowing it, and whether they are strong enough to override the presumption against excluding a potential source of organs for transplantation.

The aim here is to cover most of the arguments currently in the field of familiar debate, and to provide by implication a template for dealing with others.

The starting presumption

The methodological starting point of this whole enquiry is the claim that if life and health can be restored by transplants there is a presumption in favour of its being done, and, as long as there is a shortage of organs, against placing obstacles in the way of organ procurement. There is at least something to be said in favour of any method of getting organs—it is good in at least one way—so the question about any particular method of obtaining them can be understood as the question of whether there are objections strong

enough to overcome that presumption. Prohibition of organ selling in itself cuts off a potential supply of organs. Nobody thinks
that many of the people who would be—or are—willing to offer
kidneys in return for payment would have been likely to make
living donations anyway. In consequence, at least on the face of it,
prohibition means that people will continue to suffer and die who
might have been saved.

To repeat, this is *purely* a methodological device for getting the
argument into order—it does not settle the substance of the issue—
but it is useful in being something everyone involved in the transplant debate can agree about: an Archimedean point that nearly
every puzzled individual will be able to accept without hesitation,
at least as long as the idea of a presumption is properly understood.
And it is particularly important in the context of debates about
payment for organs, because the reaction against such payment
was so strong and so immediate that most people still tend to take
prohibition as the default position, and to presume that anyone
who wants to end prohibition needs to prove that there are positively good reasons for doing so.

In the light of this presumption, it is worth commenting briefly on
the rhetoric of the kidney-selling issue when it first came to light, and
the description of the purchasing side of the transaction as 'the
greedy rich'. Rhetorically what this does is carry the implication that
such people already have more than they need ('rich') and are furthermore morally reprehensible ('greedy'), and in doing so neatly
hides the fact that there is *anything* to be said in favour of allowing
organ selling. The language rather gives the impression that the rich
in question, tired of gold-plating their bathrooms and surfeited with
larks' tongues, have now turned to collecting kidneys to display with

their Fabergé eggs and Leonardo drawings. But although the purchasers in the original scandal must certainly have been pretty well off to be in Harley Street in the first place, they were not there because it was some luxury resort. They were there because they were in danger of *dying*, or at least trying to escape the crushing misery and accelerated deterioration of a life on dialysis. In that respect they were worse off than all the healthy people in the world.

Of course it is a standard technique of persuasion to minimize the other side of a case you are trying to make, and people who think organ selling is wrong must think that the purchasers in this case were indeed doing something morally bad. But it is essential to distinguish moral enquiry from persuasion. *Greedy* is not a word anyone would normally use to describe someone who was putting their resources into desperately trying to save their own life. It is not a word we would think of applying, say, to a friend who was travelling the world seeking out any practitioner who might offer some hope of a cure for their cancer. Of course you might, reasonably, argue that there was something wrong with a system that allowed some people to get expensive treatments like transplants when millions of people in the world were still without even basic medical treatment; but anyone who wants to pursue that line of argument would have to accept that transplantation itself should be abandoned at least for now, because it is available only to people who are, in global terms, very rich indeed. Unless the lives of the rich—people like the writer and readers of this book—are worth saving at considerable cost, there should not be a transplant programme at all.

So the starting presumption stands. If lives are worth saving by transplants, so are those of the people who try to pay for organs that would save their lives. Or at least, if their moral turpitude in trying to buy organs makes their lives unworthy to be saved, that has yet to be shown. For anyone seriously examining the issues—as opposed to going straight into rhetorical persuasion mode—the enquiry needs to start with an acknowledgement that there is a case to answer by anyone who wants to cut off this supply of organs.

Putting the issue schematically, what is needed is an argument of this form:

There is a presumption against any obstruction to organ procurement.

Prohibition of payment for organs cuts off a supply of kidneys for transplant.

But...

So prohibition should remain.

The rest of the chapter will be concerned with candidates for that '*But...*' premise. They are all familiar, appearing regularly in ordinary discussion, and in debates in the media and at medical conferences. Variations can be multiplied indefinitely, but the following discussions cover most of the familiar ground.

The main objection: harm to the sellers

Of course nobody concerned in the payment debate will, when it comes to the point, deny that it matters to save the life of someone with kidney failure. A great many of the people who are strongly opposed to allowing payment are themselves transplant or renal professionals, and perpetually preoccupied with the problem of how to increase organ donation. If they slip into rhetoric that seems to imply that would-be purchasers are so far beyond the moral pale that they are not worth saving, that is presumably because they think that buying and selling organs is so *obviously* wrong that it hardly matters what terms of moral condemnation are used. Whether or not 'greedy' is the *mot juste*, people should simply not be paying for organs. And the most commonly used argument in defence of this position is that in buying organs the purchasers—and any other people involved in the transaction—are harming the sellers. That would be the added '*But…*' premise:

> There is a presumption against any obstruction to organ procurement.
>
> Prohibition of payment for organs cuts off a supply of kidneys for transplant.
>
> *But… Selling organs is harmful to the sellers.*
>
> --------------------
>
> So prohibition should remain.

Now obviously it is horrible to recognize that some people feel they must try to sell a kidney because they are in urgent need of money. I suppose there may be some people sufficiently detached from concern for the badly off and extreme social inequality to see nothing distressing about this fact, but if there are I have never come across them. Of course it is disturbing that this should happen—just as it is when people are forced into prostitution, or health-destroying labour for a pittance, and millions of other hardships that come about as a result of poverty. That is not at issue. The question here is the *quite different* one of whether we are justified in reaching the practical conclusion that organ selling should be *prohibited*.

The immediate problem about claiming that harm to the sellers justifies prohibition is that the sellers themselves are usually willing, even eager, participants in the exchange. No doubt they are encouraged and often misled by enterprising brokers, but we know that there are many who actively volunteer, and seek out the opportunity. Consider, for instance, the case of the young Turkish father swept to everyone's television screen by the surge of outrage that followed the first revelations in the UK.[7] He was trying to meet the expense of urgent hospital treatment for his daughter, who had leukaemia. Presumably the prospect of selling his kidney seemed no more intrinsically attractive to him than it would to anyone else, but he nevertheless judged it to be his best available option. The same applies to other 'desperate individuals' who advertise kidneys and even eyes in newspapers, or write to surgeons offering to sell them, 'often for care of an ill relative;[8] or approach passing doctors to ask about the possibility. Furthermore, the interest comes not only from people in abject poverty. People in affluent countries also advertised their own kidneys on the Internet until it was made illegal, and sometimes still try to do so, or complain because they are not allowed to. Such people regard the situation they are in as one that would be improved by the money they might get, even at the cost of the loss of a kidney.

Of course there is an obvious reply to this. The sellers may think they will benefit from the transaction, it will be said, but in fact they will not. Frequent reports from campaigning organizations and investigative journalists expose exploitation, cheating, shoddy operations, lack of counselling and follow-up, and a trail of vendors

with damaged health and no lasting benefit to compensate—
frequently no better off than they were before, and sometimes actually worse off. Whether the would-be vendors recognize it or not, it
is claimed, the course they are trying to pursue is far too dangerous
to be reasonable. We, who know better, must save them from themselves for (what we hope they would agree, if they knew enough, is)
their own sakes. 'State paternalism grounded in social beneficence
dictates that the abject poor should be protected from selling parts
of their bodies to help their sad lot in life.'⁹

The argument, then, seems to be along these lines:

There is a presumption against cutting off any potential
supply of life-saving organs.

Prohibition of organ selling cuts off one supply.

The potential sellers want to sell because they also expect to
benefit.

But... *They will not in fact benefit, and may end up even*
worse off.

We should not allow them to make choices that will harm
them.

Therefore payment for organ donation should be prohibited.

The first of these added premises makes a claim of fact, about the
way the world is and how it works. The second makes a moral claim
about how we ought to behave.

The first thing to notice about the moral claim is that it is
incompatible with the principles now generally accepted in liberal
societies, and increasingly in medical contexts, that people should be

allowed to make their own decisions about what is in their own interests. The argument depends on claiming that the would-be sellers of organs should not be left to judge for themselves what is in their interests, but should have the matter decided for them by a paternalistic state. So one thing that needs to be done by anyone thinking through the issue is to decide what to think about that premise. Is it really acceptable to give up our usual liberal principles about autonomy, and allow the state to decide what is good for individuals in this context?

People who are reluctant to allow any kind of paternalism may try to get out of the problem by claiming that people who try to engage in organ selling are not really competent to make their own decisions. But if anything resembling normal legal standards of competence are accepted, this line of argument is a non-starter. Virtually all the people concerned would unhesitatingly be regarded as competent in other contexts, such as making contracts and consenting to other medical procedures—including unpaid organ donation. The non-competence claim could be reached only by counting as incompetent anyone who wanted to sell an organ, just in virtue of their wanting to do so. This may well be what is intended, but is totally incompatible with any current standards for the assessment of competence.

Anyone who wants to prohibit organ selling on grounds of protecting the sellers, therefore, cannot avoid shifting from strong principles of individual autonomy to some kind of paternalism. That is the first question that needs to be decided by anyone thinking through this issue. If you are a strong libertarian you cannot be led by a concern for the vendors to a conclusion that organ selling should be prohibited.

However, many people of broadly liberal inclinations are willing to shift to a more moderate view. Even though individuals should always be free to determine what *constitutes* their own interests, it may be argued, perhaps it may be justifiable to go against their immediate wishes if a mistaken or inadequate understanding of the facts results in mistaken beliefs about *how to achieve* those interests. Many people who resist full-blown paternalism—where the paternalist decides all aspects of what is best for someone else—nevertheless think that this kind of 'weak paternalism' can often be justified. Doctors often admit to sometimes acting without patients' consent in order to achieve what patients themselves would count as their long-term interests; and, they claim, those patients are grateful afterwards. This is the kind of thinking that seems to underlie the idea that 'since paid organ donors will always be relatively poor, and may be underprivileged and undereducated, the donor's full understanding of [the] risks cannot be guaranteed',[10] or that Western standards of autonomy are not appropriate in quite different cultures.

Suppose, then, you are willing to accept some kind of paternalism—weak or strong—and use that as the basis for reaching the conclusion that prohibition is justified. The argument now depends on the truth of the added factual premise: the claim that people who sell organs will end up no better off than before, or even worse off.

Since this is a book about the critical analysis of arguments, not about the facts themselves, I shall not discuss any of these claims about the harm that is currently suffered by organ vendors. I have no doubt that it is widespread. Nevertheless, a good deal can be said about the kind of evidence that would be needed to justify such claims. First, it is not enough to produce evidence of people who are badly off after they have sold an organ; you also need to compare their situation with what it would have been if they had not done so. Second, you need to look for evidence not only of people who have suffered, but also of others who have benefited and have no regrets. There may be many such people. Third, even when considering the ones who have suffered in some way, you need to think of their situation as a whole, not just from one point of view. For instance, suppose the Turkish father mentioned earlier had in fact been allowed to sell his kidney and his health had been damaged, but his daughter had been saved. How should that situation be assessed from the point of view of whether the person was left worse off by organ selling? Or consider a man who sold his kidney to prevent his children from being born into bonded labour. If he succeeded in this aim, it is not obvious that he would have regarded the situation as all-things-considered worse than before, even if his health suffered.

I have no firm view about any of these matters, as it seems to me that nothing like enough systematic, objective work has been done in the area. But in fact that does not matter here, because the most important point to make in this context is that nearly all the evidence we currently have is, anyway, *irrelevant*. Even if current evidence showed conclusively that vendors nearly always ended up worse off than before it would still not support the conclusion that organ selling should remain prohibited, because the harm to which these people come is *against the background of prohibition*. In other words, nearly all the evidence is about what has happened in a black market, where there can be no control over what goes on and no redress when things go wrong. This is irrelevant to the question of what would happen if organ selling were not illegal, and were subject to the kinds of standard that we automatically apply in other areas of law-governed life.

In the context of arguments about whether payment for organs should be legal, the implication of the claims about evidence of harm is that it is payment *as such* that causes harm. But living organ donation is now so safe that many surgeons actively recommend it, and they would hardly do that if they expected a string of dead or damaged donors. They expect that virtually all donors will make a full recovery to normal health. But the only obvious intrinsic difference between paid and unpaid donation is that the vendor receives something in return—which is, to all appearances, a positive advantage. This suggests that if kidney vendors are in practice disproportionately harmed, the reason must lie not in the loss of a kidney in itself, but in the surrounding circumstances. No doubt these are complex, and I shall mention other possibilities later. But it is striking that nearly all the harms alleged—cheating, careless medical practice, and lack of screening, counselling, information, and follow-up—are exactly the ones you would expect of a black market.

It probably seems as though the argument here is heading along the lines of the familiar one for legalizing currently prohibited drugs: the claim that because so much harm is done by the illegality itself, we should lessen it by legalization. But the two cases are quite different. Prohibited drugs are in themselves harmful, and there are good reasons for wanting to make access to them difficult. Making it easier to get hold of them, through legalization, would have its own bad consequences, so there is a legitimate debate about which of the two bad possibilities is the worse. In the organ-selling case, in contrast, we have as yet *no* reason to regard paid organ donation *in itself* as likely to make things worse for the vendor. Quite the opposite: if such transactions could be arranged as they might in principle be arranged, to benefit both vendors and recipients, it would be *preventing* them that did the obvious harm. As far as the evidence so far goes, organ selling, under the right circumstances, could in principle be of enormous benefit to many people.

There is, of course, some minimal risk in kidney donation, whether paid or not. Whether any risk is worth taking, however, depends on the reward balanced on the other side, and if the reward is an amount of money that could transform the life of an individual or family, it is hard to see why anyone should regard the minimal risk of a properly performed nephrectomy as not well worth taking. This chapter is being written during the financial crisis that began in 2008, and it is easy to imagine that many of its affluent-world victims might willingly sacrifice a kidney to prevent something as catastrophic as the repossession of their homes. The expected benefits should be even greater to the desperately poor, who might see in selling a kidney the only hope of making anything of their wretched lives and perhaps even of surviving, than to the relatively rich with mortgage problems. It is worth remembering, for instance, the thousands of Indian farmers who commit suicide every year because they are in debt. It is no good saying, 'They shouldn't be in this situation!' Of course they should not; but simply taking away this possibility, without offering them any alternative,*

---

* One prominent campaigner against organ selling, when it was pointed out that removing this option did nothing to provide the vendors with anything better, replied, 'That's not my problem.'

does nothing but harm. There are probably millions of people in the world who would be better off for a properly conducted, properly rewarded, properly followed-up kidney sale. In fact, if we are going in for paternalism we should recognize that the poorer you are the *more* rational it might be to risk selling a kidney. Even in cases where kidney selling might not be worth the risk in the present illegal market, a benevolent paternalist might well encourage many people in that direction if the surrounding circumstances were right.

It has been claimed that vendors come to harm even in the few places where selling is legal. But apart from the fact that the evidence for this is scanty and contested, even this is not relevant to the question of *whether prohibition should continue.* Nobody who argues against prohibition is claiming that every possible kind of system allowing organ selling would be beneficial to both sides. To argue that prohibition is unjustified is to leave *wide open* the question of what arrangements for regulation there should be if payment were not totally prohibited. It is certainly not to say that there should be a free market. The presumption against prohibition implies simply that great mutual benefit for sellers and recipients is *possible,* and that this fact provides a strong reason for trying to find an arrangement that achieves such mutual benefits.

So the argument from current harms to vendors—even to the extent that it is well supported and well researched—fails to defeat the starting presupposition against prohibition. On the contrary, the potential interest of the vendors adds to the strength of that presumption. A properly regulated exchange could in principle be as good for many of the sellers as they hope it will be, and there is no doubt that at least a large part of the reason for its not being that way in practice—either for sellers or for buyers—is the illegality and consequent lack of control. If we are concerned about the well-being of the people involved, we should be trying to set up systems to make sure that any transaction really is in their interests: arranging for regulation and supervision, committed vendors' advocates, proper legal protection and all the rest. We certainly have not yet seen anything, even under paternalistic rather than libertarian ideals, to suggest that prohibition is justified.

Of course it *might* turn out, when we started to experiment with regulation rather than prohibition, that we could not find any way to avoid a preponderance of harm over good. I shall consider that point, and others like it, in the final section of this chapter. But we cannot even do such experiments as long as prohibition continues, and we therefore have no such evidence. In the meantime, we have so far added to the presumptions *against* prohibiting payment for organs. Prohibition deprives both vendors and recipients of enormous potential benefit, and it also exposes the determined or desperate to the evils of an unprotected market that allows for no redress if things go wrong. On the face of it, the harms of prohibition are immense.

The other objections

It is important to stress that the argument so far does not show that prohibition is wrong. It shows only that *one particular line* of argument in defence of prohibition does not work; but that still leaves open the possibility that others might succeed.

It is worth stressing this point, because in spite of its obviousness as soon as it is thought about, it is surprisingly often overlooked in ordinary political argument. People defending a particular conclusion often feel impelled to defend every argument produced in its defence, and react to criticisms of particular *arguments* in defence of a conclusion as if they were arguments against the *conclusion* itself. But acceptance of a particular conclusion does not imply commitment to any particular argument in support of it, as it is easy to demonstrate. You can easily devise indefinitely many bad arguments for any proposition you regard as true.[†] The fact that claims about harms to vendors have not (yet, at least) succeeded in showing that prohibition is justified does not show that it cannot be justified by some other argument.

So far I have argued that the starting presumption, in favour of getting transplant organs for people who need them, should actually be regarded as *strengthened* by a second presumption in favour of allowing vendors to achieve potential benefit, and a third about protecting both sides from harm. The challenge is now to find a '*But…*' premise strong enough to defeat all these presumptions, and show that prohibition is nevertheless justified.

Proposals here stretch in never-ending line, and it would be impossible to cover all the variations of detail. The rest of this section covers the most familiar, and by implication shows (I hope) how to deal with others of similar kinds.

[†] For instance, along Swiftian lines, it might be argued that children should be properly fed because otherwise they will not be very enjoyable when we eat them. The conclusion (that children should be properly fed) is not defeated by the fact that the offered justification is absurd; and, conversely, someone who argued against the justification should not be taken to have argued against the conclusion.

Even this selection of them is quite long, and there is no need to plough through them all if the going gets heavy or tedious. By all means skim the headings and see which ones look plausible enough to investigate further, and leave the others out or come back to them later. However, it will be important to return to the text on p. 94. The section that begins there deals with arguments of a quite different kind from the ones that are discussed in the rest of this section, and the two need careful distinguishing. The difference is one that is usually missed in the heat of the debate, but which any serious enquirer needs to recognize.

Coercion by poverty

Arguments about ignorance and incompetence concern what might be called *internalities*: characteristics of agents themselves that would make them incapable of choosing properly among whatever options are open to them. The most familiar arguments about autonomy and consent in the organs debate, however, are of a different kind. Most depend on the idea that would-be vendors are coerced by external circumstances, and that since coerced choice cannot count as genuine, the option of organ selling should not be allowed.

The commonest agent of alleged coercion is poverty. 'Surely abject poverty...can have no equal when it comes to coercion of individuals to do things—take risks—which their affluent fellow-citizens would not want to take? Can decisions taken under the influence of this terrifying coercion be considered autonomous? Surely not...'[11] And, it is implied, since coerced consent is not genuine, kidney selling should be forbidden.

This is a familiar line of argument, still commonly used. It seems to work as an objection to the argument so far in some such way as this:

Prohibition deprives both potential buyers and potential sellers of the possibility of great benefit.

It also does great harm by exposing the desperate to an unprotected black market.

But...   *The sellers are coerced into their decision by poverty.*

Coerced consent is not valid (autonomous/genuine).

Valid consent is essential

\---------------------

Therefore organ selling should be prohibited.

It is easy to see how this idea gets going. Coercion typically involves human coercers, who reduce your options until the best one left is the one the coercer wants you to take. If some dealer in organs kidnaps your daughter and threatens to chop her up for spares unless you sign the deeds of your house away to some accomplice, of course you agree to do it—not because you want to give up your house, but because the kidnapper has reduced your range of options until this is the best one left. Before the kidnapper came you could (and obviously would) choose to keep both your daughter and your house; now you have to choose between them. Similarly it may seem, if only metaphorically, poverty coerces the organ sellers into doing something they do not really want to do. The poor do not want to lose their kidneys: they would rather have both the money and their kidneys. But poverty forces them to choose between the two, and giving up the kidney seems the better option.

Furthermore, to continue the analogy, when you have signed the documents and got your daughter back, you can go to court and try to remedy the situation. If you can persuade the judge of the circumstances under which your consent was given, that consent will be declared invalid and your house returned to you. So by the same argument, it may seem, we should regard the consent of organ sellers as invalid. Since no one sells an organ unless they are coerced into it by some kind of need, all consent to organ selling should be discounted as invalid.

But although the paradigm case of invalid consent (the kidnapping) and organ selling have in common that both involve constricted ranges of options, the resemblance is entirely superficial. Closer consideration shows that the analogy does not work at all.

In the first place, the constriction of circumstances that made your consent invalid in the kidnapping case had nothing to do with your having only a small range of options. You might be immensely rich and own a dozen houses, but that would have nothing to do with the matter of validity. The reason for regarding your consent as invalid is that it has been obtained by an *illicit* reduction of your options, designed to achieve the kidnapper's ends, and the illicit coercer must not be allowed to benefit from his nefarious activities. The metaphorical coercion involved in having only a small range of options is an entirely different matter, and irrelevant to validity of consent. This shows most clearly if you consider the *purpose* of declaring consent invalid, which is to restore or compensate for the options that had been unjustly constricted. Suppose, by way of contrast with your taking the matter to court after the event to get your consent declared invalid, the police had come on the scene while your daughter was still being held by the kidnapper, and forcibly prevented you from signing the document handing over your house. They might have had their reasons—perhaps wanting to demonstrate that kidnapping could not be profitable—but it would have been preposterous for them to give as a justification the argument that because you were being coerced, your consent was not valid. The point about the declaration of invalidity by the judge, in the paradigm case, was that it was *you* who wanted the declaration of invalidity. Since you had got your daughter back, the judge could, by declaring your coerced consent invalid, restore the range of options that had been unjustly curtailed (keeping both your daughter and your house). In the case involving the police, by contrast, the kidnapper has already curtailed your range of options by forcing you to choose between house and daughter, and now the police have come along and constricted still further the horrible range the kidnapper had left. The kidnapping would have been just as illicit and your consent just as invalid as before, but the point of declaring consent invalid, when we do so, is to *remedy* the situation, not make it even worse.

This is why it is quite wrong to say that the poor should be protected from selling their kidneys, 'preferably, of course, by being lifted out of poverty',[12] but otherwise by the complete prevention of kidney sales. Of course it would be much better to remove poverty, but putting the matter this way implies that prohibition and 'lifting out of poverty' are unequally desirable variations on the same general theme. The foregoing argument shows them to be, in the relevant sense, direct opposites. Protecting the poor from kidney selling by removing poverty works by increasing the options until something more attractive is available—and, of course, is strongly preferable. But prevention of sales, in itself, only closes a miserable range of options still further—like the police's preventing you from saving your daughter. To the coercion of poverty is added the coercion of the supposed protector, who comes and takes away what the prospective vendor sees as the best that poverty has left.

In other words, the argument depends on a straightforward confusion. Particular kinds of coercion do justify a declaration of invalid consent under particular circumstances, but those do not include the metaphorical coercion involved in having only a limited range of choices. And, furthermore, the purpose of declaring consent invalid is to remedy an injustice to the coerced individual. The supposed remedy proposed here (prohibition) just exacerbates the injustice—or at least disadvantage—that is being complained of.

To this it is perhaps worth adding that even if you could make these inferences from coercion by poverty, it could make no distinction between sales and unpaid donations. If vendors can be said to be coerced by circumstances, then so, for the same reasons, can donors. If losing a kidney is intrinsically undesirable, it is just as undesirable for a donor as for a vendor, and chosen only because constricted circumstances—someone else's imminent risk of death—have made it the best option all things considered. If coercion is supposed to be a reason for not allowing organ sales, and poverty is supposed to count as a relevant kind of coercion, this kind of coercion by threat of the death of a friend or relative—quite a heavy kind of coercion, you would think—should equally rule out donation. The logic is the same, so unpaid organ donation would have to be ruled out on the same grounds.

Coercion by unrefusable offer

A different kind of argument from the same direction is that tempting someone like the Turkish peasant with a payment of several hundred times his annual income amounts to making him an offer he cannot refuse, and coercing him in that way. For instance, it might be said that we should object to any 'externally applied constriction of an individual's right to choose not to donate', and include in this category 'all cases where a person sells one of his organs during life', because 'here the financial benefits have such an impact on the life of the donor and his family as to be irresistible: the element of voluntariness of donation must be at least compromised, or, in extreme cases, abolished.'[13]

This argument can be expressed thus:

There are strong presumptions against prohibition.

But...   *The sellers are coerced by unrefusable offers.*

Coerced consent is not valid.

\-

Therefore organ selling should be prohibited.

The first thing to do here is clear out of the way one idea that usually turns out to be lurking in the background when this particular objection is put forward. This is the idea that if you take someone who is very poor and offer them a lot of money, they become so dazzled by the prospect that they lose all capacity for judgement and make the wrong decisions. Presumably this might happen in some cases. If so, however, the argument changes: it turns into one based on incompetence to consent rather than coercion. In any situation where this was suspected you would need to do an assessment of competence on a case-by-case basis. You cannot just presume that everyone in such a situation must be incompetent.

Furthermore, when the consent given for some procedure is decided to have been incompetently given, the conclusion is not *that the procedure must not go ahead*, but only that it cannot go ahead *on the basis of that consent.* The judgement of incompetence is usually taken to imply that someone else, who is competent, should make the decision in the incompetent person's interests. This goes back to the arguments about paternalism. Even if you thought someone had been dazzled into incompetence by the offer of a large sum of money, you might still decide that the exchange, under proper circumstances, was strongly in the person's interests. So this direction of argument could not support the conclusion that there should be prohibition.

However, the argument as it stands is not about incompetence but, once again, about validity of consent. It is the mirror image of the previous objection. In this case the coercive agent is not poverty (as it were) pushing from behind, but the unrefusable offer pulling from in front. Does the idea that the resulting consent is invalid fare any better with this interpretation of coercion?

The first thing to be said here is that the first added premise is simply false. Coercion (as already argued) involves reducing the range of available options, and here what is happening is exactly the opposite. A new option is being added; and that, at least on the face of it, looks like an advantage rather than a ground for complaint. The possibility of selling a kidney means that you can choose to get money that would otherwise not have been available to you. This means that whoever is using this argument needs to explain it much more fully, since we cannot assess it without understanding what is intended.

Perhaps the idea is something on these lines. If you are a prospective vendor you do not actually *want* to lose your kidney; you are doing it *only because* of the prospect of payment. The offer of money is making you do something you do not want to do.

But if this is the idea, then, as with the matter of coercion by poverty, it is just an illusion generated by superficial associations of words. Losing a kidney is something people do not want *in itself*; so perhaps it may seem that in preventing someone from making this choice you are protecting them from doing something they do not want to do. But when the thing they do not want *in itself* has been made a part of a package with a great deal of money attached, it has become something they *do* want *all things considered*—which is, of course, the whole point of offering inducements. It would be extraordinarily perverse for anyone to claim, on the basis of a concern for voluntariness, that because you disliked one element of an attractive package your consent should be declared invalid, and you should be left in a situation whose combined elements you liked even less. If the argument seems to work, it is only because of an equivocation between wanting something *in itself* and wanting *all things considered* a package that contains it.

Another feeling may be that if the offer is impressive it leaves you with *very little choice* about whether to accept it, and if it is impressive enough it leaves you with *no choice* at all. This seems to catch the intuitions referred to earlier, about the difference between compromising and abolishing voluntariness.

However, this will not do either. It may sound plausible, but it depends on attributing a literal meaning to a metaphorical phrase, since—oddly enough—the expression 'had no choice' is never used except when there is in fact a choice. If you are asked why you jumped into a raging torrent and your choice did not come into the matter, you do not say 'I had no choice about jumping'; what you do is deny the implication that you made a choice and say 'I didn't jump, I slipped', or whatever. If on the other hand you say 'I had no choice, my child had fallen in', you obviously did have a choice, and what you mean is that the option of not jumping in was unthinkable. Similarly, if you say 'I had no choice about selling the kidney; they offered me enough money to get my family out of poverty', what you mean is that it would have been absurd for you to take the option—still open to you—of keeping your kidney and remaining in poverty. If having no choice in this sense compromised or abolished voluntariness in a way that invalidated consent, it would follow that valid consent could occur only when there was not much to choose between the available options. You could not validly consent to marry the suitor whose merits were immeasurably beyond those of his rivals: your consent to accept one of the available candidates would be valid only if they were so much of a muchness that it made no difference which you took.

This would actually be quite a useful line of argument for opponents of organ selling. It would mean that the only way to make consent voluntary and therefore valid would be to reduce the price until it was unclear that the transaction was worthwhile, and by then the deal would have become so pointless that no one would consent to it anyway. But, oddly, this is a kind of argument that people do use in many contexts. Something like it is used, for instance, to argue that if you pay people to help in risky things like medical research you must not pay *much*; and I have recently heard

68

people claiming that if payment for organs were allowed, the amount paid must be strictly limited. Arguments of this kind are presented as arising from a concern for the people who might be tempted to accept, but it is extraordinarily difficult to see how they are supposed to work. Perhaps the idea is that a small amount is not likely to dazzle anyone into incompetence; but if so, that is hardly a reason for not making an offer that a competent person would have overwhelming reason to accept. Perhaps it is that if only a little is offered, the people you attract will be the ones who are intrinsically willing to do whatever it is you want them to do; but that does not work, because the small amount might result in your getting only the people who were absolutely desperate for money.

Anyway, whatever mysterious ideas are going on in the background (I shall make a suggestion in the next chapter), it is a remarkable idea that if you are asking people to do something rather unpleasant or risky, giving them large payments is somehow going against their interests or wronging them in some way. It sounds like the Victorian idea that the pay of the lower orders should be kept down, or they would just spend it on drink. This line of argument is obviously a non-starter as a serious account of voluntariness and validity of consent. The whole point of offering inducements is to make people willing to consent to what they would not otherwise do, and the more unrefusable the inducement, the more reason there would be to suspect any *other* choice of being invalid.

These are not the only arguments about coercion in the field. It is also objected that allowing organ selling can be indirectly coercive, in exposing people to coercion by others: if the option to sell organs is there, people may be put under pressure to take it. This claim is important, as are others of a related kind, but they raise different issues. They will be discussed later.

Exploitation

An objection of a different but related kind is that payment for organs is bound to involve exploitation. Poverty may not make people irrational, it may be agreed, or invalidate their consent, but it does make them vulnerable to exploitation. The vulnerable must be protected, so prohibition should be continued.

This argument can be set out like this:

There is a presumption in favour of allowing payment for organs.

But...   *Organ buying is exploitative.*

People should be protected from exploitation.

Therefore payment for organs should be prohibited.

The first problem here lies in the way exploitation works, and, once again, the crucial difference between coercion and inducement to do what is intrinsically unattractive. Coercion works by the removal of better options until the unattractive one is the best left, and in such cases it is possible, as already argued, to protect the victim by putting a stop to the coercer's activities and restoring the original range. But exploitation does not take this form. It works the opposite way, by adding inducements until they just tip the balance, and an intrinsically unattractive option becomes part of a package that is, all things considered, the best available.

What is supposed to be bad about exploitation, and is regarded as differentiating it from the offering of inducements that is a normal part of buying and hiring, is that the exploiter seeks out people who are so badly off that even a tiny inducement can improve on their best option, and in that way can get away with paying less than would be necessary to someone who had more options available. (If this is exploitation, of course, it looks suspiciously like free market capitalism; there is nothing new in that idea.) But the fact remains that it works by inducement, and the logic of inducements still applies. Nobody can directly improve your position—*protect* you—by removing an effective inducement, however small, because to do so is to take away what you regard as your all-things-considered best option. (People may of course be deluded into thinking that some inducement is in their interest, but that is a different matter. Exploitation is often accompanied by deceit by the exploiter or misjudgement by the exploited, but it need not be.)

In other words, we have an argument with unexceptionable premises—that the poor are vulnerable to exploitation and that they should be protected from it—but whose conclusion does not follow. Although we can stop the exploitation by stopping the trade, to do so would be like ending the miseries of slum dwelling by bulldozing slums, or solving the problem of ingrowing toenails by chopping off feet. We put an end to that particular evil, and thwart the exploiters (which may be a motive in its own right), but only at the cost of making things even worse for the sufferers of exploitation. So if the concern is to protect the vulnerable, it cannot—once again—be done simply by taking away their best option. It can be done only by giving them better options.

The obvious way to do this, of course, is to compel the exploiters to give them better payment and conditions. It is interesting, however, that this obvious remedy for exploitation never seems to be suggested by people who say organ selling is exploitative; and in fact the more you recommend in the way of payment, the more it seems you are likely to attract accusations of coercion by unrefusable offer. It seems that no amount of payment could be fair; and what that means is that organ selling is being regarded as *inherently* exploitative, not just exploitative under certain conditions. In that case, however, the usual meaning of 'exploitation' is being stretched out of all recognition. It usually means something like 'taking advantage of someone's weak position to pay them less than they should be paid', or treating them badly in some other way, but in such cases there is a complete remedy in paying the right amount (whatever that is supposed to be). If *no* amount of money or care in treatment could make organ selling non-exploitative, it is clear that 'exploitation' is being used with a quite different meaning. Before we can assess the argument, therefore, we need clarification of this new meaning. We need to know what it is about organ selling that is supposed to make it *inherently* deserving of the normal negative connotations of 'exploitation', irrespective of how much is paid— so that we can then decide whether we agree with the implications. What could it be?

This is a challenge to the person making the complaint—and until it is met the argument cannot continue, because we do not know what the complaint is. (That is an absolutely serious point, not a philosophical quibble. It is a common trick of argument to describe a situation by using a word with strong negative connotations, and imply that even if the word is being used in some different sense from the usual one, the negative connotations still apply.) The most intuitively plausible interpretation is something like 'it is exploitative because the people concerned would not agree to do it if they had enough money; you are getting something you would not get if they were in a stronger position'. That is true, but there are two problems about it as a premise in an argument to the conclusion that payment should be prohibited. First, as it stands it applies to just about all paid work, and much familiar selling. Unless you would do your job for no payment (because of its intrinsic satisfaction and your not needing money), anyone who employed you or bought what you offered for sale would in this sense be exploiting you—making use for their own purposes of your need for paid employment. If that is the intended meaning, it does not differentiate organ selling from innumerable other things people would not do if they had enough money without doing it. And second, it is still difficult to see how prohibition could help anyone said to be exploited in this radically extended way. Probably the people who clear rubbish and clean drains would be doing something else if life had given them more opportunities, but it would be absurd on several grounds just to say that their doing such things amounted in itself to exploitation, and that the work in question should be banned—rather than that pay and conditions should be made as good as possible.

What seems to be happening here is something familiar in political argument: a sleight of hand that can be very effective in persuasion. A word in common use has its meaning stretched, and it is taken for granted that the stretched version can still trail the negative connotations of the original. It looks suspiciously as though 'exploitation' here is just a rhetorical device for conveying the moral disapproval of the speaker, without any specific content. If it is supposed to have content—to express some aspect of organ selling as such that supports the inference that it should be prohibited—we need to be told what that is in order to assess it.

And, incidentally, if the poor are being exploited by the rich in this case, it might equally be said that the well—the organ sellers—are exploiting the sick, by demanding the money needed to cure them. And, of course, not only the organ sellers, but the transplant surgeons whose high incomes depend on the fact that their skills are desperately needed by the unfortunate. Giving substance to rhetoric often has startling implications, which is presumably why it so often remains as rhetoric.

Altruism

The claim that organ donation must be altruistic is presented, like the voluntarism requirement, as a moral absolute overriding all weighings of harms and benefits. Financial inducements, it is said, are to be ruled out because they preclude altruism, and an absolute requirement of organ donation is that it should be altruistic.

Since this requirement is usually asserted rather than argued for, it is presumably taken to be self-evident. Nevertheless, it is surprising. At least the other arguments discussed so far have started with plausible moral concerns—about coercion and exploitation—and have foundered only in the transition between these premises and the conclusion. But in this case the principle itself, for all its supposed self-evidence, seems positively at odds with all our usual attitudes. The world is, after all, full of transactions that the transactors see as being to their mutual benefit, and to which in principle we have not the slightest objection. We may particularly admire their one-way equivalents, when goods and services are given and nothing is expected in return; but it normally does not occur to us that unless some transaction can be guaranteed to be of this one-way kind it should not take place at all. It would normally be regarded as astonishing, and in the absence of pretty impressive justification absurd, to claim it would actually be better that neither side should benefit (neither vendor *nor* recipient) than that both should.

Even if we accepted this remarkable principle, however, it would still have the now-familiar problem of not supporting the required conclusion. Altruism is about motives: doing something with the aim of benefiting someone else rather than yourself. (It is also a matter of degree: a matter of the *extent* to which you sacrifice your interests to someone else's. So an altruism requirement would have to specify the threshold of sacrifice required to qualify.) But you cannot control people's motives by making rules about what they are allowed to do. You can, of course, try to arrange society in ways that encourage altruism, and make people generally inclined to think of others rather than just themselves, but the rules and institutions organize what is possible, not people's motives for making choices. And, quite apart from that, there is no necessary connection at all between payment and non-altruism or between non-payment and altruism. If a father who gives a kidney to save his daughter's life is acting altruistically, then so, by the same criterion, is one who sells his kidney to be able to pay to save his daughter's life. If it is altruistic to work long hours to earn money for your family, it is altruistic to sell your kidney for the same purpose. Conversely, if you donate a kidney because you are hoping your uncle will change his will, or because your entire family is making your life miserable by bullying you to donate, you are not donating altruistically.

So even if there were any justification for holding as a principle that organ donation was unacceptable unless altruistic, it would still not support the prohibition of payment. In fact the only way to get from an altruism premise to the required conclusion would be by *defining* 'altruistic' as 'without payment'. There are some contexts in which the contrast between giving and selling is described as between doing things altruistically and doing them for payment, even though this is not the general meaning of the term. If this kind of contrast is thought of as paradigmatic, the demand for altruism may get its apparent force from seeming to coincide with the absence of payment, while at the same time giving the appearance of offering justification because nobody doubts that altruism is a good thing.

The altruism requirement, in other words, looks suspiciously like a mere restatement of the non-selling requirement, with spurious moral knobs on. If so, the argument is straightforwardly question-begging. It amounts to claiming that since it is a fundamental moral principle that organ donation should be unpaid, it should be unpaid.

Human dignity

The issue of question-begging definitions arises also in the context of another common claim: that organ selling is incompatible with human dignity. This idea appears in both the WHO statement[14] and the Declaration of Istanbul[15] mentioned earlier, and the claim that we should respect human dignity itself sounds beyond debate. But to assess this claim as an argument in defence

of prohibition we need to know what human dignity is supposed
to consist in, so that we can see first whether we accept that particular account, and second whether the non-selling conclusion
follows from it.

The problem is that no account whatever is usually given. Like
the altruism requirement, the dignity requirement is usually just
asserted; and if we know no more about human dignity than that
it precludes organ selling, the argument is once again question-
begging. You cannot use a concern for human dignity as a justification for opposing organ selling if you have no better explanation of
what dignity is than that it rules out organ selling. So we need a
non-question-begging account of human dignity, as applied to
these questions, before we can assess this argument.

The WHO statement does attempt an account: it claims that
payment for organs 'conveys the idea that some persons lack dignity, that they are mere objects to be used by others', which is presumably intended to reflect the Kantian idea that people must not
be treated merely as means to other people's ends. But paying
people for goods and services is not generally regarded as treating
them as mere means. In fact, the involvement of payment—as
opposed to enslavement or force—shows that what is going on is a
transaction between two consenting people. So that does not
work.

Futhermore, I should have thought that most people's conception of respecting human dignity, these days, would include as an
essential aspect allowing them to decide for themselves what
counted as good for them. The last thing human dignity seems to
call for is telling people who are badly off that they cannot be
allowed to try to improve their situation because some paternalist

thinks it is in some vague way better for their dignity to remain as they are.

More will be said about this matter of dignity in the next chapter.

Slavery

(It is perhaps worth adding a reminder that if these arguments seem to go on for ever—as indeed they do in practice—and are getting tedious, you should skip to p. 94 or just read any parts of this section that look particularly interesting. It can always be returned to later.)

Another argument, frequently produced as decisive, is that selling body parts is like slavery. Everyone now agrees that slavery should not be allowed, it is claimed, so they should by parity of reasoning agree that selling parts of people is also wrong.

I find it a straightforward mystery that this claim is so common. As in the case of coercion by poverty, an argument by analogy depends on the closeness of the analogy, so we need to see whether any of the things that are objectionable about slavery are also found in selling parts of yourself. I suppose the idea must be that buying a part of someone is rather like buying the whole person, but if this is the idea it is a pretty remarkable one. If you buy or sell a slave, you are treating another person—who should be regarded as an autonomous human being, not property—as something belonging to other people, to be passed from hand to hand as they please. But to draw an appropriate analogy with selling a kidney you would need a circumstance where *someone else* was the owner of your kidney. If you decide to sell your own kidney it has nothing to do with anyone else's owning you. The very fact that it is yours to sell presupposes that you are the one in control of what happens.

It may be said that this does not help because it is not just other people who cannot sell you into slavery; the law does not allow you to sell *yourself* into slavery either. But if that is the idea, there are two things wrong with it. First, the law against slavery is not actually stopping *you* from doing anything. If you choose to live and act as somebody else's slave, nobody will stop you; all the law says is that the other person may not imprison you or force you to do anything, and that it will refuse to enforce any contract you make allowing yourself to be treated in that way. The restrictions on slavery apply to the entitlements of potential owners, not to the behaviour of willing slaves.

But, more directly to the point of the organ-selling analogy, the law is not just about *selling* yourself into slavery; it applies just as much to *giving* yourself (or anyone else) into slavery. And here the appearance of any analogy with the organs case breaks down entirely—because what is puzzling about the objection to allowing payment for organs is that they can legally be given. You are entitled to make over something of yours to the sole use of somebody else, as long as you are not paid. The whole problem centres on why something which is ours to give should not be ours to sell. Even if the slavery argument worked in other respects, it would not begin to provide an answer to this part of the problem.

Commodification

A similar common claim is that organ selling should not be allowed because it commodifies the body.

This claim is true by definition, because having monetary value, and being transferable between people on that basis, is exactly what a commodity is. But then the question remains of what is supposed to be bad about it. The word carries strong connotations of disapproval, presumably rooted in our horror of treating people themselves as commodities, but before the moral implications can be dragged over—before we approve the loaded word 'commodification' in this context—we need to see whether the moral suggestion is justified.

As the slavery argument shows, it is not. Once again, treating people as commodities, with no say in their own destiny, is just about as different as it could be from letting them decide for themselves what to do with their own bodies or parts of them. This is what is at issue here, and it might reasonably be regarded as the most fundamental of all matters of autonomy.

Ownership

Another variant on the slavery and commodificiation arguments concerns ownership. It is often argued that we cannot sell our bodies or parts of them because we do not own them.

The first question to ask of anyone who produces this argument is about the status of the claim about ownership. It may be intended as theological: a claim that our bodies belong to God. In that case the matter would have to be discussed with the relevant theologians, and the obvious first point to raise with them would be that you cannot usually *give* away what does not belong to you, either. Not many religious people seem to object to unpaid kidney donation.

But even if there were a clear answer to that objection, it would be irrelevant to the discussion here. The conclusion to be defended is that payment for organ donation should continue to remain illegal, which would mean the argument had to be along these lines:

Bodies are owned by God; we do not own our bodies.
It is against the will of God for us to sell our bodies.

Therefore organ selling should be prohibited.

Unless you put into the argument a premise to the effect that civil law should reflect divine law (of the kind recommended by the arguer), the conclusion does not follow. Most people reading this book probably think that the law should as far possible allow religious people to follow their own consciences (in this case, refuse as individuals to buy or sell organs), but that no specifically religious constraint should be imposed on everyone. (This matter will be taken up again in Ch. 5.)

Another way to interpret the non-ownership premise would be as a claim about current law, and if so, it correctly reflects the fact that bodies do not legally count as property.[16] However, although the premise is in that sense true, the conclusion does not seem to follow, even within existing law. We can give organs to other people; and if that does not count as a transference of ownership, but as the provision of a service, there is no justification for not describing payment for organ donation in the same way. (And, of course, there would have been no need to prohibit payment for organs if it had been ruled out by existing law.)

Anyway, the existing state of the law is irrelevant to the intended conclusion of this argument, which is about what the law *should* be. Even if there were some reason to think that only property could be paid for, that would still leave the question of whether we should change the status of transferable body parts to count them as property. Most people now think we should have the right to decide whether to *give* our kidneys, and the right to give normally implies ownership. If there is a good reason for claiming that we should have a kind of legal ownership that extends to giving but not selling, it is, to say the least, not obvious what it might be. I shall return to this matter later.

Benefits to the rich

Another common claim is that allowing organ sales is wrong because it gives benefits to the rich that are not available to the poor. The argument sounds attractive because it appeals to an egalitarian principle, but it runs straight into problems. In the first place, virtually nobody would be willing to defend, when pressed, a principle to the effect that unless everyone can have some benefit, no one should. Since the *essence* of being rich is having access to benefits that the poor have not, this would amount to a demand for absolute economic equality; and though there are some people who advocate this, it is not a claim that often appears in the transplantation debate.

A modified version of the idea might be that the rich should not be able to get privileges of specifically health-related kinds that are unavailable to the poor. But although many people are concerned about inequalities in health, there are very few who would accept the implications of a claim as strong as this one. It would rule out not only all private practice in medicine, but also all the advanced treatments routinely available even to the relatively poor in parts of the developed world with universal medical services. As already commented, transplantation itself is almost exclusively a privilege available only to the people who are—globally speaking—rich, so obviously nobody involved in the transplant debate can accept this argument. And if they did, they should be campaigning for the abolition of other health privileges available to the rich—including free medical treatment for the relatively poor in rich countries.

Even if they were willing to accept the premise and its implications, however, it would still not support the conclusion. It might support a prohibition on the *private* purchase of organs, but it would be irrelevant in contexts where the purchaser was some public body, buying organs to distribute impartially to its population. Once again, it is important to stress that claiming that prohibition is unjustified implies nothing at all about what arrangements should be in place if the absolute ban were removed. Many people who are not opposed in principle to payment for donation think that the only acceptable arrangement would be purchase by public bodies for distribution on the basis of need. This has been suggested by various commentators,[17] and happens in Iran. Even if the premise were acceptable, the conclusion would still not follow.

Targeting the poor (Istanbul)

The objection that organ selling is wrong because it targets the poor is not one often encountered in ordinary debate, but it is included here because it appears in the highly influential *Declaration of Istanbul on Organ Trafficking and Transplant Tourism*, which has already been mentioned several times. The familiar assertion about human dignity appears as an objection to trafficking and tourism, but the only argument for prohibition of payment for organ donation ('transplant commercialism') that appears in the document is that '[b]ecause transplant commercialism targets impoverished and otherwise vulnerable donors, it leads inexorably to inequity and injustice and should be prohibited'.

Since this Declaration has been so widely endorsed it is worth commenting a little more generally on its contents. 'Organ trafficking' is defined in terms of cheating, deception, exploitation and the like.[18] Of course it is a good thing to draw attention to the extent to which this goes on, and to exhort transplant practitioners to be on the lookout for it, but it is a rather surprising topic for a Declaration, since nobody would think of disputing the unacceptability of practices of this kind. (It seems unlikely that anyone would put out a Declaration against Murder—unless of course murder, perhaps of a particular group, had become regarded as acceptable.) But the Declaration also rules out 'transplant tourism'[19] and 'transplant commercialism',[20] and the presentation of all three in the same context conveys the impression that there is some essential connection between them. The implication seems to be that if you are against one you should be against the other two as well.[21]

Now of course at present, because payment for organs is so widely illegal, many actual instances of paid donation are likely to involve something reasonably described as trafficking. But it is essential to recognize there is no *necessary* connection between the two at all. In other contexts it is quite clear that the wrongness of trafficking is quite irrelevant to the question of whether the same activities would be wrong if the elements of cheating and force were not present. The fact that the trafficking of migrant labourers is bad and should be stopped does not begin to suggest that employing workers from overseas is itself wrong, let alone that employment of all kinds is wrong. In the same way, the wrongness of trafficking organs shows *nothing whatever* about the wrongness either of allowing payment for them, or of allowing paid transactions between countries. If these other things are to be shown to be objectionable, therefore, that needs separate argument, not just an imputation of guilt by spurious association with trafficking. But the only argument against allowing payment in the whole document is the one quoted above: that it 'targets impoverished and otherwise vulnerable donors' and 'leads inexorably to inequity and injustice'.

This is another case in which substance must be distinguished from rhetoric. 'Targeting' implies taking deliberate aim, and in this case, by implication, malevolent aim. (It is obviously not intended to imply targeting the poor for receipt of some benefit.) It suggests the sort of thing that is done by loan sharks when they deliberately seek out people in need because they are most likely to be susceptible to what they have to offer; and no doubt the same is true of many organ brokers in the present black market. So the use of the term already carries strong negative connotations about the motives of anyone involved in transplant commercialism. But removing the prohibition on organ selling—or failing to establish it in the first place—does not involve picking out any group at all, let alone picking it out for bad treatment, and certainly does not imply malevolent intentions or self-interest. There is no targeting of any kind involved.

Of course, it can often be claimed that even if some law or its removal is not *aimed* at a particular group it nevertheless *affects* some groups more than others—though if this is what is intended the term 'target' is entirely out of place. So, would allowing payment—removing prohibition, or failing to establish it in the first place—adversely affect the poor? That is what remains when the targeting claim is recognized as rhetoric.

The first point to make is that the people affected by allowing payment for organs would not just be the poor. The as-it-were targeted group would be the people who would want to buy or sell organs if payment were allowed, so it also includes all the people who are sick and could be saved by a kidney if they (or their health providers) were allowed to buy them, as well as all the people who would sell if they could. Although undoubtedly this second group consists mainly of the very poor, we also know that many among the relatively rich would be willing to offer a kidney if they thought it worthwhile for the money they could get.

And second, what the rhetoric implies is that these groups would be *harmed* by allowing payment for organs. It is said that payment 'leads inexorably' to inequity and injustice. It is not clear whether this is supposed to mean 'inevitably produces' or 'inevitably involves'; but either way, if this were to be anything more than another piece of rhetoric—if it were to be used as part of a serious debate—it would call for not only a good deal of empirical evidence, but also careful explanation and justification of this use of the rhetorically useful but analytically slippery terms 'inequity' and 'injustice'. Nothing of the kind is offered. And, as argued at length already, removal of prohibition would not *harm* the 'targeted' groups. In principle they could all benefit from properly controlled, legal, paid donation. If they are affected in a bad way, as the rhetoric implies, it is *prohibition* that targets them, not payment itself. They are harmed by being prevented from doing what could be good for them, or exposed to harm if they risk illegal arrangements.

Any appearance of justification for prohibition in the Istanbul Declaration comes from the spurious association of the harms of trafficking with the putative harms of allowing payment as such, the implication that selling must always harm people who are already badly off, and, for good measure, the rhetoric of 'targeting'. There is no argument whatever here, only smoke and mirrors. For a major international statement, widely endorsed, this is appalling.[‡]

Persisting black markets

When it is claimed that the harm to the sellers is done by uncontrolled transactions, rather than by selling in itself, it is often replied that even if we made legal, controlled selling possible, it would still be impossible to prevent black markets. The desperate—both for kidneys and for money—would therefore still be driven to them.

That is almost certainly true; and it is worth commenting in passing that this fact would present a serious problem for the organization of legal arrangements for payment. The high safety record of organ donation comes largely from careful screening of the health of donors; but the more stringent you made the safety requirements for legally controlled arrangements, the more potential vendors would be rejected, and the more would find

---

[‡] I know very little of the politics in the background of WHO and Istanbul. As far as I know, however, no moral philosopher known to have argued in detail against prohibition was invited to the latter.

their way to the unprotected black market. How best to handle this problem would present real problems for attempts to organize legal arrangements.

However, although the claim itself is true, there remains the question of what people who raise this point (as many do) think can be inferred from it. How is it supposed to fit into the debate about legalizing payment? This an important point to insist on in debates in general, where disputants are usually more inclined to argue about the truth of each other's claims than what could be inferred from them if they were true. The matter of relevance is the fundamental one, because if nothing of any significance would follow from the truth of some claim it may be irrelevant to consider whether it is true or not.

This is a challenge for anyone who makes the claim that black markets would persist, and I have never heard it met. However, we can consider various possibilities. For instance, how would it fare as a 'But…' premise in the familiar argument?

> Both vendors and recipients could benefit from a properly regulated system of payment for organ donation.
>
> But…   *An unregulated black market would persist anyway, harming both.*
>
> --------------------
>
> Therefore we should continue to prohibit organ selling.

If this looks at all plausible, consider some analogies:

> Both our country and overseas workers could benefit from a properly regulated system of immigration.
>
> But…   *People would still organize illegal immigration, harming both.*

So we should prohibit all immigration.

Or, during the debates about legalizing homosexuality in the 1950s:

Homosexuals would have a much better life if their activities were not illegal, leaving them vulnerable to arrest, persecution, and blackmail.

But... *Some people would still persecute and blackmail them, in spite of the law.*

So homosexuality should remain illegal.

These other illustrations make it clear that there is no connection at all between the premise that objectionable illegal forms of a legal activity will always go on and the conclusion that we should make or keep the activity itself illegal.

In particular circumstances, widespread law-breaking may be used as evidence that the public does not support the law in question, and as part of an argument that it should therefore be *repealed*, as for instance when the laws about suicide were changed; and the fact that so many people do currently engage in illegal buying and selling of organs, by mutual consent and with direct harm to no one else, might well be part of the argument for repealing current laws against it. But it could not possibly provide a justification for prohibition in the first place.

My guess is that what is intended by people who produce this line of argument must be something like this:

Some people want to end the prohibition of payment for organs.

They justify this by claiming that doing so will end the black market in organs.

But there would still be black markets outside any legal market.

So there is no justification for ending prohibition.

If this is the intention, it is probably already clear where it goes wrong, at least as an answer to the lines of argument developed in this chapter. To start with, limiting the harm of black markets is not offered as *the justification* for ending prohibition (see the contrast drawn earlier with the argument about legalizing drugs on p. 55). The fundamental justification is that allowing mutually beneficial exchanges is presumptively good for both sides. Black markets are brought into the argument only as a reply to the people who try to defeat the presumption by claiming that allowing payment does harm: most of the harms alleged to result from allowing payment in fact result from the black markets that are the inevitable result of *prohibiting* payment. But even if limiting the harm of black markets had been offered as the main justification for ending prohibition, as opposed to an additional benefit, it would still be irrelevant to point out that black markets would still persist alongside legal markets— which nobody doubts. The fact that we cannot protect everyone, because some people will always break the laws whatever they are, is hardly a reason for not trying to protect anyone.

It is crucial, in all serious debates and enquiries, to consider where claims that are made are supposed to fit into the argument as a whole. Often a claim that is true may nevertheless be irrelevant.

Better ways of doing things

When it is claimed that prohibition deprives two sets of people in great need from making a mutually beneficial exchange, one common response is that this is still not the right way to go about remedying the situation of either group. What we should be doing is lifting the poor out of poverty, and doing far more to persuade people to donate.

This, like the rhetoric about the greedy rich and the exploited poor, is persuasively powerful in conveying the impression that the dispute here is between people who think that organ selling is a perfectly good way for the poor to get out of poverty ('enthusiasts' for a 'trade', as I have often heard them labelled), and their idealistic opponents who think there are better ways of running the world. But this is why it crucial to keep the subject of the debate clear at all times, and why the argument format can be so useful.

Of course it would be better in many ways not to take organs from living people (paid or unpaid, for that matter), and of course it would be good if everyone were so well off that kidney selling could not possibly benefit them (though I find it hard to imagine such a situation). But nobody is claiming that organ selling is an intrinsically desirable practice, and that is not the question at issue. The question is whether organ selling should remain *prohibited*. If the 'better ways of doing things' response to organ selling is to be regarded as relevant to this question, it would have to fit into the arguments in some such way as this:

Prohibition deprives the poor of a way of improving their situation.

But...   *We should be lifting the poor out of poverty!*

So we should continue to prohibit organ selling.

And

Lives could be saved if selling kidneys were permitted.
But...   *There are better ways of getting organs!*

So we should prohibit organ selling.

Merely expressing the arguments in this way is enough to show why they do not work; in fact it is hard to see how they are intended as arguments at all, as opposed to *cris de cœur*. It is not that there is anything wrong with the added premises, which nobody would be likely to dispute. It is just that, as in the arguments of the previous section, as they stand they have no obvious connection whatever with the required conclusion.

In the first place, in both cases the claim that some other situation would be better cannot possibly count as a reason for acting as though that better situation already exists. Even if we should be working towards improvement in both matters, that is not at all obviously a reason for preventing people from making the best of the less good situation in which they currently are. Nobody is suggesting we should be recommending organ selling *rather than* trying to reduce poverty in other ways.

And second, whatever the actual situation, arguments on these lines could not possibly work for logical reasons. If people were well enough off not to want to sell their organs, or if there were enough donated organs to supply the need, there would be no *point* in prohibition, because nobody would want to buy or sell. There is no point in prohibiting something that nobody wants to do. Conversely, if prohibition does achieve anything, *precisely* what it achieves is preventing the people who might benefit from buying and selling from doing so. In other words, in the ideal situation (no poverty, no organ shortage) prohibition is pointless, and in the less-than-ideal situation we have at the moment (poverty and organ shortage) it does harm. Either way, it is unjustified.

The only obvious way to repair the logical structure of these arguments would be to add another premise, to the effect that allowing sales would actually *impede* the alleviation of poverty and the development of other ways of getting organs, along these lines:

Prohibition deprives the poor of a way of improving their situation.

But... *We should be lifting the poor out of poverty!*

Allowing kidney selling would actually make it harder to alleviate poverty.

So we should continue to prohibit organ selling.

And

Lives could be saved if selling kidneys were permitted.

But... *There are better ways of getting organs!*

Allowing kidney selling would actually discourage donation.

So we should continue to prohibit organ selling.

Claims of this kind are indeed frequently made when the inadequacy of the first attempt at this kind of argument is demonstrated. This turns them into a quite different kind of argument, which needs a separate kind of discussion.

This is what now follows.

A different kind of argument

The arguments listed in the previous section (from p. 58), with all its subsections, have been what might be called one-liners: they claim that we must not allow payment for organs because doing so would directly contravene some existing, generally accepted principle. I have argued that all these arguments fail for one reason or another. Either the premises do not support the conclusion (as in the arguments involving exploitation or invalid consent), or the principle invoked is one its proponents would not accept in other contexts (the altruism requirement, the unacceptability of privileges for the rich), or the principle has no clear content at all (human dignity). No doubt there are variations on these arguments that have not been dealt with here, but these represent most of the ones in familiar circulation. ('Circulation' is, incidentally, the right term: they go round and round, starting again when they reach the end. I shall return to that matter in the next chapter.) It seems unlikely, at this stage, that organ selling in itself can be shown to contravene directly any of the familiar principles and values that underlie our normal ethics and politics. On the contrary, all our usual values, such as saving life, respecting autonomy, allowing mutually beneficial exchanges, and protecting everyone from harm, still provide a strong presumption in favour of removing total prohibition.

If any of the arguments of this kind had worked—if allowing payment for organs could have been established as being in direct contradiction to some principle that was generally regarded as beyond question—it would have followed that prohibition was justified. However, *the converse is not true*, and this is an extremely important matter—not just for this debate, but for all parts of practical ethics. Even though organ selling does not in itself directly contravene any of the moral principles that underpin our social organization, it might still be argued that in *practice* prohibition nevertheless reflects the best balance of good and bad that, in a messy world, we can see how to achieve. Even if there is nothing that justifies its being ruled out immediately and directly, there might still be reason for thinking that prohibition would, on balance, be the best policy.

Arguments that take this form appear all over the organs debate, generally in the form of assertions about harms that would occur if payment were legalized. The pervasive claim about harm to vendors (pp. 48 ff.), for instance, comes into this category, though it was not there identified as different from the one-liners in the following section. But suggestions about kinds of harm are potentially endless: 'mutual respect for all persons will be slowly eroded',[22] or '[organ selling] invites social and economic corruption...and even criminal dealings in the acquisition of organs for profit';[23] or payment 'undermines altruism'[24] (though it is not clear there whether the claim is meant to be that payment constitutes lack of altruism, or whether it is thought to spread a kind of selfishness through society), or 'leads to profiteering and human trafficking',[25] or that if purchase is a possibility, related donors are more reluctant to come forward,[26] or that there will be no incentive to overcome public resistance to a cadaver programme.[27]

The difference between ruling out some policy in principle and deciding that it would not be good on balance is sometimes expressed as the difference between giving moral and *pragmatic* reasons for reaching some practical conclusion; but that is misleading. If you want to argue that some arrangement is best in practice you are still implicitly depending on criteria for deciding when one set of outcomes is better than another, and the question of what criteria should be used for that purpose is itself a moral question. So-called pragmatic judgements involve *both* empirical claims about the way the world works *and* moral claims about which values we should use to compare different possible arrangements. What this means is that although this kind of reasoning—about how to produce the best outcome, and which risks we should take—is something we do all the time, it is in theory immensely complicated. It is quite different from judging *directly* that some policy should be recognized as wrong.

In practice the difference between the two kinds of argument is not usually recognized at all, and most arguments in passionate debates slither around between the two kinds. It is essential to distinguish them, however, because arguments of this second sort need a completely different kind of analysis. In particular, they usually cannot be dismissed on the basis of logic alone in the way I have argued that the many of the one-liners can, because they depend so heavily on empirical claims. This may be why they seem to be increasingly popular, as the arguments of principle are shown to run into trouble.

When people do assert in these ways that some harm would result from the removal of prohibition, they often seem to think that the case for prohibition can be regarded as proved unless their opponents can prove their claim wrong. This, however, would be a mistake. The failure of the arguments of principle in the previous section leaves the original burden of proof intact—and indeed much stronger, by now, than the minimal starting point launched in the Introduction. A justification is needed not only for reducing the supply of organs, but also for preventing both buyers and sellers from achieving great benefit, and exposing them to the risk of positive harm. This means that anyone who wants to produce an argument of this kind needs to make the case out *positively*—not just presume it stands until the other side has produced a conclusive refutation of it.

The problems of doing this were to some extent indicated in the earlier discussion of harm to the vendors, but these can be generalized and expressed as wider principles of rational enquiry. Such principles show that assertions about harm that would come from ending prohibition can never be accepted, just as they stand, as reasons for overcoming all the presumptions in the other direction.

First, if you were genuinely considering whether to implement some policy such as prohibition, and started with the recognition that there was a presumption against it, you would not dream of implementing it because of the mere *possibility* of harms that might ensue. A serious enquiry calls for a careful risk analysis, involving identifying and weighing possible goods and harms and assessing the probability that each would come about. This involves empirical research, ideally involving experiments and pilot studies—and it is (once again) highly significant that the current prevalence of prohibition makes such research impossible. If an argument of this sort is to be taken seriously the first thing it needs is real evidence. It is at this point that the argument about harm to the vendors fails. We have no reason to think, a priori, that selling must in itself harm the vendors, and nearly all such a posteriori evidence as there is comes against a background of illegality and inadequate control, and is therefore largely irrelevant.

Second, as also discussed in the context of harm to the vendors, it is not enough just to establish the likelihood of harm that would result from the removal of prohibition. It is also necessary to assess the loss of benefit on the other side, and engage in moral debate about the relative merits of the two. This is an enormous undertaking in large-scale contexts, and anyone producing an argument of this form needs to demonstrate at least having taken the matter seriously.

Third, the appropriate response to real evidence of probable or even certain harm, in contexts where there is a presumption in favour of some policy, is not a rush to prohibition but serious efforts to devise ways of keeping the good elements while avoiding the bad. Nearly everything we do—including trade of all kinds, and of course such ordinary activities as driving or flying—carries potential for harm, but it does not usually occur to us to abolish the whole thing rather than try to lessen or remove its dangers. When we do have such an impulse it usually means that we really regard the activity in question as bad in itself, and are using the alleged dangers as an excuse to oppose it. As already mentioned, this is the kind of reply appropriate to claims about harm in contexts where some research has been done into controlled organ selling—in Iran and the Philippines, for instance. The results of this research are at present very far from conclusive either way, but to the extent that they do show harm, the challenge should be to find other ways of arranging matters that avoid it. If the presumption against prohibition is taken seriously, it should be regarded as a last resort.

Could a satisfactory argument against all organ selling, of this more complex kind, involving balancing good and harm, ever be found? It would have a lot of hurdles to clear, but it certainly cannot be ruled out. For what it is worth, my guess is that the most promising kind of argument along these lines would be related to the fact that there are many contexts in which it makes good sense for people to want to have particular options closed to them. It is too simple to presume that giving people a new opportunity must necessarily count as an extension of their options in any relevant way.

The reason why it can often be perfectly rational to prefer not to have certain choices open to you, even though you would take them if they were available, is that keeping some options closed may be the best way to achieve what is more important to you at a deeper level. Most people know from their own experience what it is to choose to keep out of the way of temptation of various kinds, even in such small ways as not keeping biscuits in the cupboard because they would eat them if they were there. In the same way, it is easy to imagine contexts in which people might prefer not to have the organ-selling option open to them in case their family started to bully them into selling, or they were tempted to use kidneys as guarantees for loans, or as stakes if they were compulsive gamblers. There are obvious dangers in making organs too much like other possessions. The economist Robert Frank[28] also suggests why societies deliberately limit the role of money, and resist allowing payment for body parts. He points out that a good deal of what individuals strive for is the improvement of their *relative* position. Someone might sell an organ to get ahead of their competitors, but then the competitors would be under pressure to do the same to catch up, and then everyone would be minus a kidney but in the same relative positions as they started from.[29] (You may be able improve your view by standing on tiptoe, but if everyone stands on tiptoe the view is the same as before and they are all worse off.) These are seriously interesting considerations, because they show how issues of autonomy—what people actually want for themselves—can lead to a willingness to close certain options.

But even if such arguments are produced and substantiated, there are still various methodological points that remain relevant to any serious enquiry.

First, there is still a presumption against prohibition: you would need positively good reason to accept it because it still, certainly, does various kinds of harm. There are many people, both potential vendors and potential recipients, who could benefit enormously if the option were available, so there would still be a requirement to try to prevent the harm to some people without also cutting off the benefits to others.

Second, an argument that depended on claims of fact in this way would be permanently susceptible to revision in the light of change in either evidence or the facts themselves, so even a well-supported conclusion that prohibition was justified could not be regarded as permanent—as it might be if it breached a point of fundamental principle. It should therefore remain permanently under review, with the presumption against it remaining in place.

For this reason it is vanishingly unlikely that such an argument would work for all times and all places. If some argument of the kind just outlined were to work, for instance, I would expect the conclusion to apply within particular groups rather than universally.

Furthermore, if the justification were to be in terms of autonomy rather than paternalism, the pressure for restrictions should come from within such groups themselves, rather than being imposed by external paternalists.

There is more evidence now of serious enquiry into different ways in which payment for organ donation might be implemented than there was ten years ago, and various people have made serious attempts to think of ways to allow the good aspects of kidney selling while lessening possible harms.[30] But still, most of the arguments alleging its dangers are put forward as if they provided justification for total prohibition, and are accompanied by no suggestion of willingness to experiment or devise ways of limiting harm. There is very little evidence of concern with systematic empirical enquiry among most of the advocates of absolute prohibition.

This leads to the subject of the next chapter.

3

METHODOLOGICAL
MORALS

This chapter is more theoretical than the others, so anyone who wants to concentrate on the practical issues can go straight on to the next chapter—perhaps skimming the last two sections of this one before doing so. Similarly, anyone who starts and then finds it heavy going should give up and move on. But I hope anyone who does this will eventually come back. The content is important, because the book is about the harm that can be caused by mistakes in moral reasoning, and I discuss here how some of those mistakes occur.

The form of the arguments

Because ethics in practice is so commonly thought of as a top-down activity, which starts with moral principles and then applies them to particular situations as they arise, it is important to emphasize the form the arguments so far have taken.

It often seems to be taken for granted that anyone who is against total prohibition of payment for organs must be a strong libertarian who thinks that individuals should be left to make their own judgements in a totally free market. But although it is true that extreme libertarian principles do entail some such conclusion, the converse is not. The arguments of the previous chapter do not depend on libertarian principles at all, and they do not reach the libertarian conclusion that there should be a free market in organs. In fact they do not depend on any substantial political or moral theory whatever, or reach any positive conclusion about what policies and arrangements there should be about payment. The starting point of the enquiry is the absolutely minimal claim that there is a presumption against total prohibition, and the conclusion is the equally minimal one that this presumption still stands. This conclusion merely *opens up*, rather than settles, the question of what kinds of restriction and regulation there should be—*including*, possibly, in some places and at some times, a total ban.

In the normal run of political debate, where opposing sides are bent on achieving their ends by whatever means they hope will be effective, arguments about policies get mixed up with allegations about the character and motives of people who support them, and, as already commented, the issue of organ selling is often presented as if it were between 'enthusiasts' for a 'trade' in organs, who can see nothing to dislike about the idea, and their morally concerned opponents who are determined to protect the poor against the rapacious rich. But, in fact, the arguments here have not depended on any disagreements about values and attitudes at all.

It is clear, for instance, that no opponent of organ sales would dispute the starting point of this enquiry, that it is intrinsically good to save lives by transplants when we can. They must therefore also accept the claim—when properly understood—that as long as we are short of organs there is always a presumption in favour of getting more, and that no possible source should be rejected without good reason.

That might suggest that the disagreement between the two sides was about what constituted good reason, and that differences of moral approach would show up at that point. But very few of the objections raised here to the familiar defences of prohibition have disputed the moral premises on which those arguments are based. I have not denied, for instance, that freedom and autonomy are good things, or that people should be protected from exploitation, or that slavery is wrong, or that valid consent is essential for organ donation. What my arguments have claimed is that these principles simply do not support the required conclusion.

In one or two places I have disputed the proposed principles themselves—as in the case of the mysterious altruism requirement, or the claim that the rich should not have benefits denied to the poor. But in those cases it is it is clear that even the proponents of the arguments themselves do not generally accept the principles offered, because they would reject their implications in other contexts. Anyway, even if they did accept them, there would still be the problem of their not supporting the conclusion. In other cases the problem is that it is not clear even what the relevant principle is supposed to be. Until the appeal to human dignity is given more substance, for instance, the argument amounts to nothing but a question-begging reassertion of the conclusion, and cannot even be discussed.

So the arguments offered here have not depended on any appeal to controversial moral principles. Nor have they depended on controversial empirical claims. Even in the cases where empirical claims are used to defend prohibition—all the claims about harms suffered by the vendors, for instance, and indefinitely many others about wider harms to society—the only reply made here has been to outline perfectly general, surely uncontroversial, principles about the way rational arguments of this form should work. So, for instance, evidence collected against the background of a black market, even if carefully enough assessed in its own right, is likely to be irrelevant to the question of what might happen under regulated conditions. And when there is, as in the case of this argument, a clear burden of proof, there needs to be positive evidence, not the mere possibility, that the predicted harms will occur and be great enough to outweigh the benefits. There should also be continuing positive efforts to find ways of avoiding any harm without preventing the good.

In other words, the attempts to justify total prohibition fail not by the alien standards of some external critic who is making rival empirical claims or offering different bases for moral judgement, but in terms of moral and intellectual standards normally accepted by *the proponents of prohibition themselves*. The arguments simply do not support the required conclusion, or they depend on principles or methods of argument that their proponents themselves do not accept in other contexts, or they depend on empirical claims for which there is nothing like enough evidence, or they are vacuous. The criticisms given here depend only on logic and analysis, and work *within* the moral and intellectual systems normally accepted by the people who are putting forward the arguments.

The significance of the failures

The next significant point about the failures of the familiar objections to allowing payment is that they are not of an obscure kind, discoverable only by deep philosophical analysis, but involve mistakes that no one would be in any danger of making in less fraught contexts. This becomes apparent as soon as the arguments are suitably transposed.

It is claimed, for instance, that concern for the vendor's autonomy demands the prohibition of organ sales, because the decision to sell involves coercion by poverty. But if you had cancer, and had to choose between some pretty nasty treatment and imminent death, nobody would for a moment suggest that because you had been coerced by the cancer into making an intrinsically unwelcome choice, your consent to the treatment should be regarded as invalid and you should be left to your fate. It is also claimed that vendors cannot give valid consent because they are coerced by unrefusable offers. But if you reluctantly came to the conclusion that you must sell some treasured family heirloom because Sotheby's had predicted it would fetch thousands of pounds at auction, thereby preventing the repossession of your house, no one would think it anything but a joke if friends expressing concern for your autonomy stole it to save you from yourself, claiming that the unrefusable offer precluded your true consent.

Much the same applies to the rest of the arguments. It is argued that organ sales must be stopped because of exploitation and shoddy practices; but if the only shop in a neighbourhood has been getting away with exploitatively high prices, or the only hospital with substandard treatment, it does not occur to anyone that simply closing them down, leaving no services at all, is a useful way to protect the local population. Or it is asserted that organ giving must be altruistic; but although we admire altruism, and are full of approval when ageing parents are looked after by their children for love, we are not usually tempted to infer from this that people who have no children, or who are not loved by them, should do without care altogether rather than have paid help. Or it is said that organ selling involves unreasonable risks for the poor, but no one thinks twice about leaving relatively well-off people to their own devices when they decide to take on risky jobs like diving from oil rigs for high pay, or go in for dangerous sports for fun—with far higher risks and much lower potential returns than organ selling. And so on.

This suggests what is really going on. The familiar arguments against organ selling are rationalizations of something already believed for other reasons. No one starting innocently from the beginnings of these arguments could possibly arrive at the conclusion to which they are supposed to lead. Their proponents are already, independently, convinced that organ selling is wrong and should not be allowed, and the arguments seem plausible only in the light of that conviction.

This is also suggested by many other aspects of the debate. It appears, for instance, in the speed of reaction to the discovery that payment for donation was going on, and in the terms in which it was immediately condemned. The outright condemnation came before there had been any time at all to consider how our usual moral principles should apply to this new phenomenon, and without any anxious weighing of pros and cons. If people had really been trying to *work out* whether prohibition was justified or not, they could hardly have overlooked so completely the obvious prima facie harms of prohibition—dismissing the people who needed organs as greedy, or somehow thinking they had helped the Turkish man who now had no way to pay for life-saving treatment for his daughter—and would have been agonizing over the complexities of the problem rather than rushing into action.

It also appears in the way every demolished argument is immediately replaced by another, with ever weaker ones recruited to the cause as the early contenders fail. As John Stuart Mill says in another context:

> For if [an opinion] were accepted as a result of argument, the refutation of the argument might shake the solidity of the conviction; but when it rests solely on feeling, the worse it fares in argumentative contest, the more persuaded its adherents are that their feeling must have some deeper ground, which the arguments do not reach; and while the feeling remains, it is always throwing up fresh entrenchments of argument to repair any breach in the old.[1]

The organ-selling debate could hardly demonstrate this phenomenon more clearly. If the first justifications offered for prohibition had been the real reasons underlying its immediate implementation, there would not have been such determination to find alternatives when those were shown to be fallacious. The people offering these arguments would simply have changed their minds.

It is also suggested less directly in many other aspects of the debate. It often appears in the way assorted arguments of quite different and often incompatible kinds are heaped up together—as, for instance, when it is complained that vendors are exploited (paid too little), that they are coerced by unrefusable offers (paid too much), and anyway should be altruistic (not paid at all). It also appears in the rapid invention of convenient facts intended to justify the policy in an indirect way when the direct arguments seem to be getting into trouble—which is also something that regularly happens when deep feelings are being defended. It is probably the conviction that allowing payment simply must be wrong, furthermore, that leads so many people (who probably know nothing of the matter) to presume that all the surgeons and clinic organizers and brokers involved in paid organ donation must be villains. There are horror stories about all these groups; but there are horror stories about all areas of commerce, and this does not tempt us to assume that all dealers must be scoundrels or all trade profiteering, or even to express outrage (as opposed perhaps to disquiet) in other contexts where vast profits are made from the practice of medicine—including transplant surgery. If it is assumed that anything earned through organ sales must be tainted, that suggests that the exchange is regarded as inherently, not merely incidentally, corrupt.

The situation, then, seems to be this. When states enact laws forbidding the exchange of money for organs, or professional bodies pronounce their anathemas against it, they present their conclusions as arising from plausible moral concerns about autonomy, exploitation, and the need to protect the vulnerable. If the criticisms offered here have been right, however, this cannot be what is actually going on. The pattern of argument shows that there must be a deep and quite independent conviction that organ sales should not be allowed, into whose defence has been a pressed a motley array of arguments that could not have begun to persuade anyone who was really trying to work out the rights and wrongs of the issue from scratch. What seems to be doing all the work here is a direct intuition, quite independent of, and fuelling, the curiously bad arguments offered in its support. The question now is what to make of this intuition.

Strong moral feelings

Everyone is familiar with the phenomenon of rationalization, which is what goes on when we try to find plausible justifications for what we already believe or want for other reasons. We do it all the time. In particular, we seem to be very good at justifying in terms of generally accepted moral principles things we really want for personal, selfish reasons, so that we can appear to others—and probably think of ourselves—in a morally acceptable light. If we do not want to give money to charity because we would rather keep it for ourselves we are likely to say—and often think—that it is because the organizers will not use it efficiently, or that foreign aid does more harm than good. If workers want to keep their jobs they are likely to argue that the jobs in question are essential to the public good. If bankers want to keep their bonuses high and their taxes low they will claim that unless this happens all the talent will leave the country.

What is interesting about the rationalizations involved in trying to justify prohibition of organ selling, however, is that these are not rationalizations of selfish motives. There is nothing self-interested about commitment to the idea that organ selling is wrong and should be forbidden. The people who oppose allowing it, often passionately, do not get any obvious benefit from prohibition or their advocacy of it. Some of them might even at some time suffer from it, if they needed a transplant and could not get one by other means. Their opposition to organ selling is genuinely *moral* in the broad sense of involving commitment to requirements that individuals think should be imposed on everyone, including themselves—even though that imposition has some kind of cost, and even when it is actually against their individual interests. The rationalizations involved here are attempts to justify a principle that is, in this broad sense, genuinely moral.

This raises the most fundamental question of all. If the moral intuition against organ selling really is so strong, and so prevalent, is that not significant in itself? Some opponents of allowing payment for body parts, when they recognize the failure of the usual lines of argument, do move into the position that Mill sees as the final retreat of his non-reasoning opponents: the conviction that their feeling reflects 'some deeper truth, that argument cannot reach'. It is often said that such strong intuitions should be our ultimate moral authority: that 'it is the emotional conviction which ultimately should determine where one makes one's stand'.[2] Payment for organs just *is wrong*.

If the wrongness of payment for organs is regarded as moral bedrock, it is indeed irrelevant that it cannot be justified in terms of other moral principles. Justification has to end somewhere, and if anyone is really determined to accept this as a fundamental moral truth it will be hard to see how to take the debate any further. If someone just asserts that they know it is wrong—that it is obviously wrong, and there is no more to be said—then certainly *argument* seems to have got as far as it can.

However, anyone tempted to sink with relief into this apparently impregnable position needs to recognize what it involves. Even though it may in itself be unassailable by logic, most people will be able to keep it comfortable only by keeping the details of their moral views unexamined, or by determined and systematic moral dishonesty.

In the first place, although strong feelings do typically appear to their possessors as compelling insights into moral truth, nobody who thinks seriously about the matter can regard mere intensity of feeling as providing the last word in matters of ethics. The idea that passionate moral feelings are reliable guides to moral truth makes no sense as an intellectual position, because, of course, passionate feelings conflict. The more committed people are to their own 'emotional convictions', the more likely they are to regard other people's as manifestations of prejudice and bigotry. Even people who insist on following conscience because they regard it as the voice of God think that religious opponents are failing to distinguish the true voice of conscience from the promptings of the Devil.

An even deeper problem is that anyone who takes the trouble to look will quickly discover that even their own moral views are full of internal conflicts. This is what I have tried to show in the case of opponents to organ selling. The slightest knowledge of history should also make everyone understand that if they had been born in another time or place they would probably have been trying to defend positions that now seem to them outrageous. The context of the Mill passage quoted above is instructive in this respect. It comes from the beginning of *The Subjection of Women*, in which Mill was trying to dislodge the certainty of most of his contemporaries that the traditional arrangements for the relationship of the sexes must be right. To us, now, his refutations of his opponents' arguments look absolutely compelling, but at the time they made hardly any headway against the deep conviction that women should be occupied in their own sphere and subordinate to men. And, exactly as Mill describes, every time he defeated a familiar defence of the status quo, more arguments—of ever-increasing absurdity—were brought in to try to repair the breaches. If his arguments look intuitively and immediately decisive to us now, that is probably because our opinions are already on his side. Had we lived a hundred and fifty years ago, most of us—including most women, since this is about morality (again in the broad sense) rather than self-interest— would probably have been scrabbling around trying to defend the traditional position of women.

Those are general problems about the idea that strength of conviction is enough to show that some moral view is right; but there are also further problems for anyone holding the specific view that they have reached moral bedrock in their conviction that organ selling must be wrong. In the first place, it looks as though most people are not actually willing to take this line—or at least, not until they are driven into a corner from which it seems the only way out—because if they were they would not need to engage in endless attempts to justify their opposition to organ selling *in terms of* other values. If it is claimed that organ selling is wrong *because* it is exploitative, or *because* it is not possible to give consent for it, or *because* it is too risky, or *because* it would dry up other supplies of organs, that suggests an unwillingness to accept that it would be wrong irrespective of such considerations.

And the difficulties go even deeper than that. The fundamental problem with accepting the wrongness of payment as a self-standing principle, rather than as derived from other principles, is that it also involves accepting that there will be circumstances in which its implications will *conflict* with the implications of those others, and that keeping to it will involve overriding them. This is the most important point. It is not just that prohibition of organ selling cannot be justified in terms of the requirement for consent, or concern for the badly off: it is that as a ground-level principle it is actually in conflict with concerns like these. Keeping to this principle must be treated as *more* important than saving life and health, respecting autonomy, increasing options, and preventing the harms done by the inevitable black market.

If someone is actually willing to bite that bullet, the argument is at an end—and at least we know where we are. As I have said, my fundamental aim here is not to argue for a particular conclusion, but to show the implications of various lines of argument. If someone claims, for instance, that organ selling is simply against the will of God, even though we may not understand why, and even though it implies that people must be left to die or left in poverty when this need not have happened, it is clear that the argument has come to an end. But in practice this does not usually happen, and the arguments just keep going round and round—back again and again to the idea that the vendors have not really consented because they have no choice, or that in practice they always end up worse off, or that the whole thing is wrong because it targets the easily exploited. This is why it is so difficult to keep these arguments in order. But to hold the moral bedrock view seriously you need to be able to confront the contradiction and still hold that prohibition is *more important* than avoiding the harms it causes. This, it seems from the constant slipping around between different attempts at justification, most advocates of prohibition are not willing to do.

Moral seriousness

'Moral' and 'ethical' are tricky words in many ways, and far too flexible in familiar usage to be worth trying to pin down with definitions. But one thing that is important is to distinguish between contexts where these words are used to express moral *judgements* and where they are used simply *descriptively*. If we claim that our country has an ethical foreign policy, or deplore the immoral behaviour of politicians, we are expressing moral judgements of approval or disapproval. If we say that some other group has quite different moral standards from ours, or that standards of medical ethics have changed in the last twenty years, we are not, in doing so, making any judgement at all, just describing states of affairs.

When we use moral words in this second way, descriptively, we are describing the standards themselves, not things that may be judged by reference to such standards. Different moral standards form the basis of different moral judgements, which means that in describing the standards themselves as moral we are not expressing approval of them. It is impossible to approve of all moral standards, because they are incompatible with each other: according to some of them, actions and policies are right or acceptable that according to others are wrong. In describing them all as moral, therefore, we seem to imply that they have something in common that makes them all moral *in kind*, in spite of their supporting different moral judgements. Philosophers have made various attempts to catch what this common factor is; and they have more recently been joined by moral psychologists, such as Jonathan Haidt, whose interest is in the deep capacity of our species for holding, following, advocating, and enforcing standards that are not in our individual interests, and may often go against them. Some such account seems to catch the idea of morality in its broad sense, and a capacity for morality in this sense certainly seems to be a characteristic of our species.

Of course individuals vary enormously in sensitivity of conscience—the extent to which they internalize their moral views—as they do in most species-typical characteristics. Some people are influenced by moral concerns only to the extent that they need to appear to conform to what others expect; others apply moral constraints to their own conduct much of the time but often give in to self-interest and feel varying degrees of guilt when they do; yet others would go to the stake rather than do what they regard as wrong. Presumably some such variation is to be found among the people who have a moral objection to organ selling. There are no doubt many who are sincere in their opposition to allowing payment, but might succumb if the person they most loved desperately needed a kidney; there are presumably others who would die rather than buy one, or let their family starve rather than sell one. There can be no doubt not only that the objection to organ selling is, in the broad sense, moral in kind, but also that many of the people who hold this view are perfectly, even passionately, sincere in their commitment to it. To that extent, and in that respect, they are deserving of moral approval.

However, to say that opposition to organ selling is moral in this descriptive sense, and to accept that most of its proponents are morally sincere in the sense of acting according to their convictions, is to say nothing at all about whether the view itself is a morally *good* one. People who sincerely believe that homosexuals should be executed and adulterers stoned, or that women need ritual purification after childbirth or menstruation, or even that Hitler was right and that we should eliminate substandard people, hold views that are in this descriptive sense moral, and may be very serious about them in the sense of being willing to sacrifice their own self-interest to enforcing them and acting according to them. You can recognize standards as moral in kind, and their advocates as morally sincere and to that extent admirable, while still thinking that what they are doing or approving is morally bad or even appalling, because you regard the standards themselves as wrong.

Here, of course, lie philosophical deep waters. If you say that some set of (descriptively) moral standards is bad or wrong, surely you are just using your own moral standards to judge other people's? And as they will similarly use theirs to judge yours, is there anything further to be said about either of them? We know what it is to judge particular actions and policies by reference to a particular set of moral standards, but how can the standards themselves be assessed? It sounds as though we need a super-standard against which to assess the competing standards; but then, obviously, we run up against the question of whether that super-standard itself is right; and that seems to lead to a vicious infinite regress. Problems of this kind soon lead many people into doubting whether it even makes sense to ask whether one set of standards is better than another, and straight into moral relativism and scepticism.[3]

Fortunately, however, that particular set of problems can be put aside for the purposes of this enquiry. To start with, nobody who is passionately sincere about their moral views can at the same time espouse either relativism or scepticism about ethics. If you really think something matters you cannot at the same time regard it as just one moral opinion among others, between which there is nothing to choose. Certainly nobody on the prohibition side of the organ-selling debate shows any sign of scepticism about ethics. Their commitment to their views is, in itself, a commitment to belief in their rightness.

And second, even though there may be problems about saying which moral view among various competitors is *right*, the arguments given here have not depended on any such claim. They have been concerned with showing that certain *combinations* of moral views *must be wrong*, because they contain contradictions.

This is the point made at the beginning of this chapter. No external moral standards were invoked as the basis of criticism of the arguments that are commonly used to defend prohibition. All the refutations depended on problems in the *logic* of the opposing arguments: premises that did not support conclusions, incompatibility of principles with others invoked by the same people in other contexts, and standards defined in question-begging or inconsistent ways.

Whatever else a set of ethical standards is supposed to do, it must provide a standard for judgement of actions and policies and attitudes, and to the extent that it is incoherent it cannot. At any point of conflict it gives opposing instructions. You cannot at once judge that organ selling is always wrong, that competent adults should be free to decide their own best interests, and that the poor should not be allowed to do what would improve their situation. However morally conscientious you are in the sense of keeping to your standards and being willing to sacrifice your own self-interest to them, if you have an incoherent set of standards you will be undermining with some of them what you claim to be trying to achieve with others. If ethics matters, it matters to be aware of such conflicts, and to try to work out what to do about them.

This suggests a quite different dimension of moral seriousness. The kind just described concerns how much you care about your moral standards—whatever they are—and how much you are willing to sacrifice to enforce and act according to them. But a deeper kind of moral seriousness concerns how willing you are to *assess* whether the standards you are so conscientiously following are coherent. These two kinds of seriousness are quite distinct. You might in principle work conscientiously to find a coherent and acceptable set of standards but follow them only lazily or when it was convenient; or you might have a seriously confused set but follow them conscientiously (but necessarily, though probably unconsciously, selectively). In particular, quite often, the more passionately serious people are about their particular moral views, the *less* willing they are to consider whether they are right or not.

Philosophers have long thought that our basic moral psychology has nothing to do with reasoning, and this is also the view of moral psychologists. We may think we reach our moral ideas rationally, and then consider how to apply them to particular situations as they arise. Really, however, we learn moral standards directly, from the people around us, and apply them equally directly. Normally it does not occur to us to reason them through, and if our moral beliefs are challenged our immediate impulse is to reach for justifications—as Mill had noticed when trying to reason with his opponents about the subjection of women—and if one justification fails we try another. When all of them seem to fail we may be (to use Haidt's term) 'dumbfounded', but we do not usually change our minds. We just remain sure that there must be a

justification somewhere, and as soon as the challenge is not immediately before us we typically slip back into our previous habits. If
this account of human psychology is right, as it seems to be, we
should recognize that the intellectual aspect of moral reasoning is
not something that comes naturally. Like our understanding and
pursuit of science, it has to be learned, and techniques must be
developed to advance it. If anything matters, however, this does.
Ethics cannot be left to simple intuition.

Rationality in ethics is not a matter of disregarding moral intuitions, but of being willing to recognize conflicts of belief and feeling and to engage with the question of which should be allowed to
prevail. The familiar arguments against organ selling systematically dodge this confrontation by trying to contrive connections
and compatibilities between prohibition and the very moral concerns that it overrides. If the arguments of the previous chapter are
right, the direct intuition that organ selling must be wrong is given
in practice the position it is denied in theory, and allowed to trump
the principles that are invoked to provide its justification. Something is seriously, objectively, wrong.

The roots of the intuition: a speculation

If you are morally serious in the fundamental sense just described,
of wanting to think through and test the moral standards you apply
in practice, what should you do when your standards run into conflict? There is presumably no general answer to that question, but
one thing that may be worthwhile in the present context is to consider the direct reaction against organ selling from a different point
of view.

The arguments in this debate—as in most debates about practical ethics—tend to be presented ambiguously between *explanations* of why opponents of organ selling feel so strongly that it should not be allowed, and *justifications* of their position. When people say why they are against allowing payment for donation, the implication is that they arrived at their conclusion because they held the moral principles to which they appeal, and were led to their opposition by the application of those principles to the case in hand. So, if they say that it is because they are against 'targeting the poor and vulnerable', or whatever, the implication is that they started with a moral commitment to protecting the poor and vulnerable, then applied this concern to the situation of organ sellers, and were led to the conclusion that payment should be prohibited. But as already argued, as one attempted justification after another is shown to fail—and to fail in ways that could not be overlooked without prior conviction of the rightness of the conclusion—it becomes clear that whether or not a justification of the policy of prohibition can eventually be found, the *explanation* of the impulse behind it must be different.

This suggests another line of enquiry. The familiar debate about whether all payment for organs should be forbidden concentrates on candidate justifications for prohibition; but if those justifications have nothing to do with the causal explanation for the feeling that there is an enormous difference between giving and selling in this context, what are the causes? Pinning them down might help to put the matter into better focus. As Mill says, the more intellectual trouble an argument runs into, 'the more persuaded its adherents are that their feeling must have some deeper ground, which the arguments do not reach'. If some other possible cause of the feeling could be identified, that might help to dislodge the idea that its only possible root must be a direct perception of moral truth.

To take a rather loose analogy, suppose you absolutely hate cats, and have for years been collecting evidence in support of a campaign to eliminate them entirely. You start with the assumption that the cause of your hatred must be your recognition of cats' intrinsic deserving of hatred. But then if you discover that you first saw a cat at the very moment when a bomb went off next to you, and your mother was terrified, it puts the matter in a different perspective. It is easier to doubt that the only possible explanation of your strength of feeling must be a direct recognition of the dreadfulness of cats. This would not in itself prove that you were wrong about them—they might actually, by coincidence, turn out to be as bad as you thought—and even if you realized that you probably had been wrong, you might still never lose your visceral horror of them. But understanding the cause of your feeling should be enough to make you question your previous convictions. It should lead you to rethink the objectivity of your collection of evidence, and at least question the justifiability of your impulse to eliminate cats entirely rather than just keeping out of their way. Much the same applies here. We know that there is something problematic about the principle that organ selling must be wrong in itself, because it runs into inconsistency with other principles that no one seems to have any intention of abandoning. But at the same time the feeling that this is not just like other cases of buying and selling is extremely strong, and it might be useful to work out what its roots might be.

Why do people—at least in Western societies[4]—seem to feel that there is something seriously disturbing about the idea of organ selling? And it is, incidentally, worth noting that the intuition is shared even by most of the people who think, as I do, that total prohibition is wrong. If I desperately needed a kidney, and none of my friends could or would offer me one, I would think in theory that there was nothing *morally* wrong with my trying to pay for one: that the exchange would make things better for both me and (I hope I would make sure) the person from whom I bought it; and that as long as everyone benefited the world would be in a better state than if the exchange had not been made. Nevertheless, I would find the whole business deeply uncomfortable. If we could work out why exactly the matter should seem so disturbing, we might be able to look whatever it was squarely in the eye and see what to make of its moral significance.

The strong revulsion apparently felt by most people is, prima facie, puzzling. It cannot be a simple, direct, learned response to organ selling itself, because when people reacted against it they had never come across it before. There cannot be an explanation along the lines of the cat and the bomb. It looks as though it must have seemed immediately and intuitively to belong to some already recognizable category of things to be resisted. But buying and selling cannot be the category, because those do not themselves provoke any such direct moral response: they are in themselves regarded as morally neutral. Nor can the removal of an organ from one living person to put into another be the relevant category, because unpaid organ donation is regarded as positively commendable. The problem is what it could possibly be about the combination of the two that produces the strong impulse to declare it off limits.

This is an empirical question of some complexity. However, since the problem is to work out what it is that triggers a particular psychological reaction—a moral horror that results in a wish to prevent whatever it is—it is an enquiry that can be started by any individual who has that reaction, by way of appropriately constructed thought experiments. As with familiar kinds of scientific experiment, you start with hypotheses about what the causally relevant factor might be, and then devise scenarios that test the hypothesis by separating this factor from other elements of the situation.

So, for instance, we might wonder whether our reaction was one of horror at the recognition of the exploitation that is undoubtedly often involved in such transactions. But in that case we should have just the same reaction whenever we consider other cases of equal or greater exploitation, and it seems we do not. When we find that third-world clothes manufacturers or coffee processors work in appalling conditions for very low pay to provide cheap goods for rich people, we may be horrified, but I have never heard of anyone whose reaction was a direct impulse to ban all garment manufacture or coffee production. Sometimes they want to close down a particular operation, but that is different from wanting to ban entirely the kind of thing it does—which is what is happening in the organ-selling case. What we say is that the people should be properly treated and paid, and that we should pay higher prices. The fact that opponents of organ selling do not do this, and usually shift to claiming that organ selling *as such* involves exploitation, shows that exploitation in the ordinary sense is not what is catching our intuitions here. It must be some other element of the situation.

Or we might wonder whether the source of the disgust was unfairness of distribution: 'wealthy people obtaining services not available to others'.[5] If so, we should feel the same immediate impulse to ban any kind of private medicine, and probably also state-financed triple bypasses for citizens of the rich world whose cost would save thousands of lives elsewhere. Again, most people will find they have no such direct reaction. And, conversely, if that aspect of the matter were removed, and organs were bought by the state for impartial distribution, that would still probably not remove most people's intuitive revulsion.

Or we might try the hypothesis that we respond differently to the two kinds of case because giving involves generosity and altruism, and selling does not. But in the first place, as argued earlier, there is no general correlation between selling and failure of altruism. A father who sells a kidney to buy his daughter medical treatment of some other kind is just as altruistic as one who gives his kidney to her directly. And quite apart from that, it is difficult to think of any other context in which the absence of altruism in some transaction leads to a reaction so strong that there is an impulse to ban it altogether—with the result that people suffer and die.

Perhaps, then, the feeling might have to do with the lack of personal connection between donor and recipient that characterizes selling: perhaps we have deep, possibly evolved, intuitions about giving parts of ourselves only when there are already such connections. But that, again, does not match the pattern of most people's feelings. For instance, the idea of so-called Samaritan donation—where living people offer kidneys to strangers—seems to generate quite different kinds of response from that of organ selling. Nor can this hypothesis account for the apparent acceptability of 'paired donations', where A wants to donate a kidney to B but is insufficiently well matched, and the same is true of C and D. If A matches

D and C matches B, the two pairs may agree to do simultaneous, crossover donations. There are now long chains of such donations, and computer programmes are being developed to facilitate them. Such donations are conducted anonymously and therefore involve strangers, but everyone seems to feel that the case is radically different from what it would be if A sold a kidney in order to buy another kidney to treat B. If so, a direct connection between donor and recipient cannot be what prompts the feeling.

Thought experiments like these make it clear to most people that when suffering and exploitation and unfairness are imagined separately from the element of selling body parts, the *direct reaction* that leads to demands for prohibition of payment for organs does not appear; and conversely, when selling is imagined with these elements absent, the feeling of repugnance obstinately remains.

These suggestions represent only the beginning of a potentially complicated enquiry; but it does seem that, over and over again, attempts to explain the objection to payment for organ donation in terms of other aspects of the situation cannot account for the response. It seems as though money as such, or comparable direct payment in kind, is itself the problem. But why, when we normally regard money as a necessary, sensible aspect of ordinary life, facilitating complex exchanges that would otherwise not be possible? Why should its involving organs make such a difference?

Here is the only possibility I have so far been able to come up with that seems to come anywhere near fitting the facts. The essential difference is that in the case of the unpaid kidney donor, the harm and risk are being accepted because a kidney is *the only thing that will meet the need*. Nothing else you could give your friend or relative would serve the required purpose, so you offer to submit yourself to the necessary harm. But if you *sell* your kidney, it has become simply a means of getting money, and anything else might in principle fulfil the same function. That is true whatever your reason for wanting the money—even saving your daughter's life.

But that itself needs explanation. Why should this fact about selling cause such a horrified reaction? The only thing I can think of is that it is because selling part of yourself looks like a desperate, last-ditch attempt to find the essentials of life. We presume that people will find any other way they can of getting money before submitting passively to the deliberate infliction of harm on their own bodies: agreeing to be mined for their own organs, as a means to getting whatever they need. Even if there is no *moral* degradation involved, submitting to harm, or seeking it out as a means to achieve some personal end, is likely (depending on context) to be regarded as a deep *social* degradation.

This suggestion needs more detailed analysis, and connection with all the work currently going on in our understanding of human nature. And since nothing really turns on whether it is on the right lines, there is no point in trying to prove the point any more tightly. It is just being thrown out for consideration. But in places where this reaction is familiar there is also much else about the debate, and the organ-selling phenomenon, that suggests that this is at least a hypothesis worth exploring.

For instance, if this explanation is on the right lines, you would expect the strength of the response to moderate as the signs of desperation got fewer. So another thought experiment might be to consider what you would feel if a comfortably-off friend chose to sell a kidney as a stepping stone to higher things: buying a bigger house, perhaps, or expanding a business. The feeling of horror should lessen, because it would suggest that the matter was more one of rational choice than desperation. If that is what most people find, it may also explain why proponents of prohibition usually imply that only the desperately poor could ever be tempted into organ selling, which is not true. The desperate situation of the people who are most likely to want to sell their organs is irrelevant to the moral question of whether organ selling should be allowed *at all*, but such cases are rhetorically necessary to produce the strongest emotional response.

The strength of the response should also moderate as the visceral perception of harm lessen. I say 'visceral' because the intuitive perception of harm in this context is probably far greater than it is likely to be in reality. For most of history, removing an organ from a living person would have been barbaric and fatal, whereas now a properly performed nephrectomy carries a very low risk of harm. But it does seem to be the case that opposition to payment for body parts and services in general varies according to the perceived harm. Nobody objects to payment for sperm donors, for instance— at least, not on grounds of concern for the donor. More people object to payment for egg donation, or surrogacy—although, as with the case of organ selling, it is difficult to disentangle horror about the real exploitation that does currently occur from objection to payment in itself. It is also interesting that many people intuitively compare organ selling to prostitution, and on this account the comparison is exactly right.*

---

* The comparison of the prostitution and paid organ donation is striking and significant. The matter of prostitution is somewhat complicated by the

The idea of degradation in payment for organs also seems indicated by the way people involved—on both sides of the transaction—do all they can to make it seem as though payment is not the essence of the matter. I have met only two kidney vendors, who were almost certainly untypical in many ways, but both of them claimed to have been motivated by altruistic concern for the (unknown, much richer) recipients, and one even said he did not

general issue of sex, which is subject to all kinds of other taboos. But our increasing understanding of sex and evolution shows how prostitution must for most of history have involved real, objective harm to women in the nature of things, not just in social convention, and therefore would usually be resorted to only in cases of desperation. Before the advent of contraception and welfare states, prostitution exposed women to real reproductive harm, both in not being able to choose their sexual partners—essentially having to take whatever came along—and in having sex without having a man committed to the support of any offspring. This is far too complicated an issue to go into here, but it is another case of submitting to harm out of necessity—or as the only means to better things—and the level of horror again seems to be connected with the degree of perceived harm. High-class prostitutes, who can be choosier about their mates and can extract a higher level of support from them, can escape the deep levels of degradation. (If this is right, by the way, it shows that the familiar feminist idea that marriage is essentially like prostitution, in connecting access to sex with financial support, is completely off the mark.) It is also significant that prostitution seems to be the only other context in which campaigners often claim that payment is *intrinsically*, not just incidentally, exploitative. It is true that most prostitution is, in practice, deeply exploitative; and, as in the case of organ selling, the harm is enormously increased by the various laws that force most of prostitution into illegality, and prevents the kind of arrangement that would lessen its drawbacks for the women involved. As with organ selling, the reaction of horror leads to a misidentification of the essence of the issue, and to legislation that makes the harm to the women involved—the really important issue—even worse. But of course this is a complex issue that needs a book in its own right, and is introduced here only to put organ selling in a wider perspective.

know about the payment involved when he first came forward—which was certainly not true. They totally rejected the idea that they had 'sold' their organs, and objected to the idea that anyone should think of the matter in that way. The impulse to minimize the significance of payment is also indicated by the fact that the relatively few people who advocate payment are inclined to describe it as a matter of 'gratuity', or 'rewarded gifting'—which seems intended to convey the impression that the action is performed out of good will, and the money is merely incidental and an acknowledgement rather than a motivation. The few people who want to arrange legal programmes of paid donation are also very anxious to find ways of showing respect to vendors, and acknowledging the value of what they are doing in the same way as with unpaid donors, which suggests an intuitive recognition that this is where the problem lies. People who regard organ selling as wrong in principle regard all this redescription and euphemism as a fudge, which from their point of view is quite right; but if the real issue is degradation the euphemism makes very good sense.

The hypothesis also suggests organ vendors in societies with the relevant values would be rather ashamed of resorting to it, and inclined to hide it. People hide things that indicate degradation. I would also predict that this inclination would lessen in people who had made a real success of the outcome, and perhaps that they would even start to boast about it—like people who are proud of their enterprise in pulling themselves out of poor origins in other ways. (This was true of the two vendors I met.)

The idea of degradation also seems to fit in with attitudes to harm and risk. As I suggested earlier, many people who claim that organ selling should be banned because of the risk to the vendors do not think twice about the rich who take up dangerous sports for pleasure. Perhaps it is also relevant in the case of people who take up certain kinds of dangerous jobs for high pay—like being steeplejacks, deep sea divers, or bomb defusers. If these jobs in themselves involve demonstrations of skill or physical prowess, the people who engage in them can be seen as embracing dangers that other people might be incompetent to attempt, rather than as people who are submitting to risky treatment by others because they are desperate. From the status point of view there is a great difference between heroically embracing danger and passively allowing other people to harm you in return for payment.

I wonder, too, whether this hypothesis may also explain the otherwise baffling determination some people have to insist on keeping payment low when it is for such things as body parts and services, or taking part in medical experiments. What low payment does is make clear to everyone that these are volunteers whom you are compensating to some extent for their help, rather than desperate people who are taking the risks because they need the money—and whom you may therefore be thought to be exploiting.

Finally, here is another kind of suggestion, even more speculative, that may be connected with different attitudes to organ selling in different societies. My suggestion here has been essentially that the reaction to organ selling is something like disgust at the recognition of degradation; but in cultures with a largely Christian background it may be harder to recognize such a reaction for what it is. The underlying system of ethics—rooted in conscience rather than shame—encourages us to think that we should fear nothing but *moral* degradation. Social shame is extremely real, as is disgust as a response to degradation, and everyone knows it; but Christian moral theology at least traditionally held that as long as you did the right thing you should not care what anyone thought about you. (Compare this with women being told that they should not care about their looks because men worth having would value only their character.) What this means is that if we directly perceive something as mattering, and want to endorse this feeling, it must somehow be translated into recognizably moral terms.

Perhaps some of the failed justifications of prohibition might be understood as gropings in this direction. 'Human dignity' is the most obvious case in point. There is indeed a loss of dignity if you are so close to the edge of a decent life that you feel you must (as it were) cannibalize your own body to survive, but what the human dignity defence of prohibition does is turn the intuitive recognition of this (descriptive) fact into a moral wrong perpetrated by other people. The altruism argument may be another such case. Somehow a suitable distinction must be drawn between the people who give their organs and the people who sell them, and 'altruism'—which has the advantage of both being flexible in usage and carrying recognizably moral connotations—can be manipulated to give the impression of doing it.

If these speculations are anywhere near the truth, they do at least fit familiar moral ideas to the extent of recognizing something seriously bad about people being in a position where selling organs seems to be a necessity. We might have just taken it for granted that it was appropriate to use the lower orders, or castes, in this kind of way—in the way most people think it is appropriate to use animals—and even if we found the idea disgusting the response might just be to keep such people and their activities out of sight. At least when it is expressed as horror that anyone should be in this position, the feeling of disgust appears as a recognizably moral concern. As one surgeon said at a conference, 'I don't want to live in the kind of society where people have to sell their organs to live.'

The problem is that there is no direct inference from morally uncomfortable feelings to morally defensible actions and policies. Undoubtedly the phenomenon of organ selling—or incentivized donation, or rewarded gifting, or whatever else you want to call it—gives many of us deep feelings of moral discomfort, especially in present circumstances where most of the people involved are in considerable need. But if we allow the feeling to direct our actions, the immediate effect will be that we try to get rid of whatever causes the feeling. If it is not reliably connected to anything that ought, morally, to be eliminated, the *only* systematic benefit of removing its cause will be the elimination of the feeling as an end in itself. This is, of course, a great advantage to everyone who suffers from it. Prohibition may make things worse for the Turkish father and other desperate people who advertise their kidneys, as well as for the sick who will die for lack of them; but at least these people will despair and die out of sight, in ways less disturbing to the affluent and healthy, and the poor will not force their misery on our attention by engaging in the strikingly repulsive business of selling parts of themselves to repair the deficiencies of the relatively rich.

And that, of course, is where the moral problem lies. None of us should want to live in a society where people need to sell their organs to live, but prohibition does nothing whatever to lessen that need, or that of the people who are dying for want of transplant organs. All it does is achieve a state of affairs where people who have such needs are not allowed to try to improve matters for themselves—at least without exposing themselves to all kinds of risks that make their situation even worse. It may be bad to live in a society where people really do need to sell their organs, but it seems still worse to live in one where they cannot do even that because the rich and healthy make themselves comfortable by prohibiting this conspicuously unpalatable manifestation of poverty and sickness, and by endless rationalizing to keep the contradictions in their moral systems out of sight. The price for such moral comfort is paid by the very people who are the supposed objects of moral concern, and it is too high. This is why serious ethics cannot be left to intuition.

Moral reasoning in practical contexts

Now let me bring together some of the elements of this chapter and the previous one, to make a general point about moral reasoning and public controversy. This involves a crucial distinction between debates about *policies or actions* that are under consideration, and debates about what *constraints* or *limits* should be imposed on those considerations from the outset.

It will probably help to start with a mundane illustration. Political and moral passions make it difficult to see the details of how arguments are working, and dull illustrations often help to make things clear.

Suppose some friends are coming to visit, and you are trying to decide which of the local restaurants to take them to.

1. You have a recollection that your guests do not like Indian food, so you start by eliminating all the Indian restaurants from consideration. You accept this as a *constraint* on the range of available options. This constraint determines one aspect of the eventual

conclusion you will reach: the chosen restaurant will not be Indian. It also determines several aspects of your initial enquiries. You will not bother to investigate the merits of the local Indian restaurants.

2. Then you find out directly from your friends that your recollection was mistaken, and they do like Indian food. That removes the constraint and opens out the possibilities again. You widen your enquiries to investigation of all the local restaurants. When you come to the end of your deliberations you may still decide on a non-Indian restaurant, for other reasons. But your former mistaken belief about your friends' preferences will have been completely eliminated as an influence on your decision.

3. Another possibility is that your friends say that they would love to go again to the Lebanese restaurant you took them to when they visited you last, and you agree to arrange that. What that amounts to is accepting an *extreme* constraint on your choice of restaurants: one so strong that it actually determines the outcome. It may be a bit odd to describe this as a constraint, but the logic is the same: the question is what you rule out before you start the detailed weighing of possibilities. In this case what you do is start by ruling out all other possibilities.

4. Suppose your friends arrive before you make any plans at all, and you are all discussing where to go. They express no preference about the type of restaurant, so you are starting with no constraints. But then you notice something odd about the discussion. As you are going through the various possibilities you begin to realize that every time an Indian restaurant comes up they start expressing doubts of quite general sorts. (Won't it be particularly crowded on a Saturday? It's close to the main road, won't it be noisy? It looks as though there's unlikely to be any parking there . . .) But they do not

seem to be raising these objections for other restaurants that might seem equally open to them; and you gradually understand that although they have not actually said they do not like Indian food, they are *in fact*, in their own thinking though not explicitly, working on the basis of a constraint that excludes Indian restaurants. They are looking for problems that will persuade you on *other* grounds to go for a restaurant that they would enjoy: trying to rationalize their preference in terms that will persuade you without revealing theirs. They may not even realize themselves that that is what they are doing. Either way, however, their non-Indian preference skews their assessment and presentation of other evidence.

In each of these scenarios the aim is to reach a practical decision (where to go), and the cases illustrate the process of making the decision against the background of different *constraints*: no starting constraint (2), a non-Indian constraint (1), a constraint so strong that it determines the outcome entirely (3), and, finally, a constraint that is not explicit and may not even be recognized (4), but whose driving influence can be inferred from inconsistencies in the discussion.

It is also important to notice that you could, in principle, reach the same practical conclusion in any of these scenarios. The Lebanese restaurant might be the best all things considered if you worked with no constraints at all (2); it might be the best non-Indian restaurant, and so would come out top if your friends expressed a non-Indian preference (1), or just worked in practice with one (4); or it might be the one your friends remembered from last time, and which you accepted as determining the outcome (3). The same *policy* might be reached for different underpinning reasons, by people who started with different constraints. So even in

(3), where the constraint determines the outcome, the constraint and the policy conclusion should be recognized as distinct, and potentially needing separate debate.

Now, in the light of this illustration—quite dull enough to prevent the intrusion of any emotions that might distort more important debates—consider, first, some general points about moral reasoning in practical contexts, and second, how they apply to the topics of the previous chapter.

If you want to reach a practical conclusion, and you are working through the problem systematically, what you should ideally do is start by deciding whether there are any constraints you should feed in at the outset. These may actually determine the policy (as in case 3 above); and even if they are less powerful than that, they may limit the possibilities you will consider as you try to reach your decision (as in case 1).

Sometimes we are clear from the outset of policy debates about the principles we believe we should accept as constraints. So, for instance, if there is a public debate about the criminal justice system in a democratic country, it is likely to start quite explicitly with principles such as a presumption of innocence and the right to a fair trial. This means that if someone comes along with evidence about (say) how much we could reduce crime by spotting dangerous 6-year-olds and preemptively incarcerating them, most people will say the proposal should be ruled out directly, and be quite explicit about their insistence on keeping certain fundamental rights for everyone. This does not mean that these principles can never be reviewed, but it does mean that as long as we accept them, they will affect the policy discussion from then onwards, and rule out some possible policy conclusions from the start. This is why it is important to make them explicit.

Sometimes such starting constraints are explicit in discussions of organ procurement policy. For instance, in most legislatures it is illegal to kill people, or cause them serious harm, even with their consent. This means that in practice most debates about organ procurement take place against the background of these principles as accepted constraints, ruling out from the start living donations that would seriously damage health (as with a second kidney) or kill (as with a heart). Of course people do challenge these underlying principles, but if they do that as part of the organ procurement debate it is clear that they are attacking a fundamental presupposition, rather that continuing the debate within the established constraints, and the two kinds of discussion are recognized as separate. It is also clear that if the constraint is removed, the discussion of procurement policy will become radically different in many ways. In countries where euthanasia is allowed, questions will arise of how, if at all, it might be combined with organ donation. In others, there will be little practical purpose in such discussions until a separate decision has been made to allow euthanasia.

In contexts like these the presence of a constraining principle may be evident and explicit. But in other cases—especially when technology has pulled us into unfamiliar terrain, and we are confronted by possibilities that are not ruled out by existing principles—something similar may be happening without our recognizing what is going on. We may *in fact* be working on the basis of strong feelings that act as constraints on the debate, but without recognizing that this is what we are doing (as in case 4 above). The most striking indication that this is likely to be happening comes when rapid, immediate, judgements are made about potentially complex questions, because those cannot usually be settled quickly unless they are regarded as being entailed by some compelling principle. When this happens it is methodologically essential to identify the existence of such implicit principles, and address directly the question of whether they are acceptable as starting constraints in the policy debate. If they are, that settles the policy issue, or at least curtails the range of possibilities to be entertained. If they are not, it is still possible that a similar policy conclusion might be reached for quite different reasons. But recognition of the difference between these two kinds of argument is essential, first for an intellectually *and therefore morally* serious enquiry in the first place, and second for a proper understanding of the status of whatever conclusion is reached. Conclusions reached as a matter of principle will change only when the principle itself is rejected or modified; all-things-considered policy conclusions will remain highly sensitive to circumstances and evidence, and as such always open to revision.

The long organ-selling discussion in Chapter 2 exemplifies all this, which is why it was important from the point of view of methodology as well as in its own right. In the real-life debate on organ selling—which might be regarded as a paradigm case of Confused Noise—the policy conclusion that payment should be prohibited is usually reached immediately, as a matter of direct moral judgement. Then, when *ex post facto* justifications start being offered, they usually make no distinction between the two kinds of argument: between defences of constraining principles that would lead to a direct rejection of organ selling at the *beginning* of the enquiry into whether there should be a policy of prohibition, and arguments that would lead to reaching the same policy conclusion at the *end* of the enquiry, as an all-things-considered conclusion. In practice the attempted justifications fall over each other in unsorted confusion:

fresh entrenchments of argument, of any kind that looks as though they might have some chance of working, are brought in to repair breaches in the old. But a properly conducted enquiry must distinguish between the two kinds of justification; and the familiar defences of prohibition can be classified in essentially this way.

Arguments of the first kind are considered in the previous chapter (in the section entitled 'The other arguments', pp. 58–94). These are the ones described earlier as one-liners: arguments intended to rule out organ selling directly. They try to show that allowing organ selling as a policy can be ruled out on the basis of generally accepted principles, such as the requirement for valid consent, and if any of these attempted justifications worked it would indeed justify a policy of not allowing payment for organs. I have argued, however, that all these attempts fail outright. If I am right in reaching that conclusion, it means you can coherently accept the principle that organ selling is wrong in itself only by recognizing it as more important than all the principles in terms of which it is usually defended, and accepting that it should override these others when it comes into conflict with them. It seems that most people are not willing to do this, which is why the attempts to defend prohibition in terms of more familiar principles continue.

The arguments given in that section, however, were only against the implied claim that ruling out payment for organ donation should be accepted as a matter of *principle*: a limiting *constraint* that should determine the outcome of the policy debate from the outset. And even if am right in claiming that all these attempted justifications fail, that does not show that the same policy conclusion cannot be reached on other grounds. The debate about the *policy* does not end with the refutation of the *principle* of non-selling. Prohibition of payment might still turn out to be the best policy all things considered.

What is important, however, is that the debate at this point should radically change its character. The situation is now like the one you are in when you find out your friends do like Indian food after all (2). We still need to reach a conclusion about policy, but the *constraint*—in this case the idea that organ selling is wrong in principle—has been removed and has become irrelevant to the policy debate, so the possibilities are wide open again. *This means that the question itself should be reformulated.* The original question is (or rather, should have been understood as) 'should organ selling be rejected at the outset *on principle?*' ('Should we rule out Indian restaurants from the start?') But the new question is quite different. It is something like 'What policies would best deal with this new phenomenon of organ selling?' ('Which of the local restaurants would it be best to go to?') And if the removal of the principle against payment for organs is taken seriously, *there is no need even to mention the issue of banning payment altogether* at this stage, even though it is possible that this might be reached as a policy conclusion. You should just consider the things you regard as mattering, like protecting people from harm and exploitation, while bearing in mind the possibility of benefits for many—in the open way that you would consider things like ambience and quality of food and parking in the restaurant case. You should work on the basis of the enquiry outlined in the final section of the previous chapter, taking great care to assess impartially any empirical evidence and its relevance, and working on a general principle of trying to achieve as much as possible of the good while preventing the harms.

What this means is that the debate about organ selling should be recognized as falling into two distinct parts. The first is about whether organ selling should be ruled out from the start as a matter of principle. The second, about which detailed policies to adopt, will then depend on the conclusion reached in the first. If in the first part of the debate the conclusion has been reached that organ selling is wrong in principle, and should be accepted as a constraint on detailed policy discussion, that will in itself lead directly to the policy conclusion that it should be prohibited. But if the constraint is not accepted, that leaves the policy discussion *wide open*. It should be as uninfluenced by the idea that organ selling is intrinsically wrong as your consideration of restaurants would be if your friends had no objection to Indian food.

This is what *should* happen. In the organ selling debate as it actually is, however, the distinction between a *starting constraint* and a *policy conclusion* is not even recognized. The debate is simply seen as one about policy, with no real understanding of the different kinds of argument that can in principle support the same policy. As a result the phase change that should occur in the debate, once the *principle* against organ selling has been removed, does not take place. People who make an immediate judgement against organ selling remain convinced that 'their feeling has some deeper ground, that argument cannot reach', and move seamlessly on from what are actually attempts to justify a *principle* that would rule out organ selling, to arguments intended to justify the same *policy* conclusion. (This is like the case of the friends who did not say that they wanted to rule out Indian restaurants from the start, but hunted around for other arguments that would lead to the same conclusion.) And if the aim is still justification of a policy conclusion reached directly, rather than an enquiry into what the policy conclusion should be, there are likely to appear all the mistakes of argument outlined in the final section of the previous chapter: treating possibilities as facts, selecting or inventing convenient evidence, and above all doing everything possible to find a justification for prohibition— rather than trying to devise ways of achieving as much as possible of the good that might be achieved by allowing payment for donation while curtailing the dangers.

It is, incidentally, worth noticing the relevance of this for debates of pro-and-con format in general. Everyone involved in transplantation will have encountered 'Paid Donation – For or Against?' debates at conferences. These never distinguish between questions of principle and all-things-considered questions of policy, and therefore just about always amount to Confused Noises. And, furthermore, the 'For or Against?' format is a misleading representation of *both* parts of the debate. Many people are indeed *against* organ selling as a matter of principle, but that does not mean their opponents must be *for* in the sense of thinking the whole thing a positively good idea ('enthusiasts'): they are simply not against on principle. And, in what should be the second part of the debate, the issue is not for or against anything. It is about which of indefinitely many possible practical policies would be the best to implement. The pro-and-con format skews the whole debate from the outset.

What needs particularly careful attention in a serious enquiry is the power of immediate, direct, judgements to stretch into the debate even when they have officially been given up as starting constraints. Even when people recognize in theory that there is no justification for opposing payment for organ donation on principle, for instance, and accept that a modification of total prohibition is needed, a close consideration of the ensuing debates will often show that, in practice, the direct judgement of wrongness is still getting in and corrupting the arguments. In particular, this immediate reaction tends to hide itself in a presupposition that even if payment must sometimes be allowed, it must be seen as an aberration, to be surrounded by caveats and underlain by the implication that the burden of proof remains on the other side.

So, for instance, consider one proposal put forward by people who had (reluctantly) conceded that prohibition could not be justified as an absolute principle.[6] They suggested that payment for donation should be allowed only among certain populations, and even then hedged round with qualifications and restrictions. 'For ethical acceptability potential kidney sellers must justify their desire on the grounds of "indirect altruism" and potential buyers must be considered for the additional social obligation of "mandated philanthropy" [essentially a tax to pay for transplants for members of the class from which the vendor came]—the decision being taken by a panel of society representatives.'[†] Because dogma is being loosened and good causes supported, a proposal of this kind may sound liberal and benevolent, but the fact remains that purchasers and vendors are to be put through a series of hoops for which no justification is offered, and that the ones who stumble

---

[†] Contrast this proposal with other things that such panels might do, such as checking for informed consent and proper conditions of sale and treatment, offering financial advice, and so on.

are left with the same unjustified harms as before. No justification at all is offered for insisting that vendors should be made to prove altruistic intentions, rather than be allowed to judge their own best interests, or why there should be a tax on this surgical procedure, and this trade, but not others. Pretty obviously, there is still lurking in the background an assumption that the whole business is inherently shady, and that if it has to be allowed at all it must be severely restricted and purified by being forced to do other kinds of good. The feelings of repugnance are still working as hard as ever to distort the analysis, and the apparent concessions only slight lessenings of unjustified harm.

The same thing shows, even more subtly, in the proposals that have been put forward for 'ethical' markets in organs. The very fact of expressing the matter in this way carries the implication that the as-it-were default market is intrinsically unethical—which, as argued in the last chapter, is not the conclusion we would reach on the basis of an extension of our normal principles about buying and selling to the new phenomenon of organ transferability. The result is that such proposals—while certainly defensible to the extent that everything they permit is in itself unobjectionable—may still curtail more good than they need to, by implying that buying and selling of organs would need to meet some such criterion to be acceptable. Even a group of transplant professionals with whom I personally have been working, specifically concerned to formulate policies that allow offering incentives for kidney donation, has come out with a proposal full of restrictions for which no justification is offered—including, for instance, that there should be a specified limit to how much could be paid to any vendor. That is, the proposal was in effect (certainly not explicitly) working on the basis of conceding that some transactions of this kind might be allowed, rather than recognizing that, given the direction of burden of proof, the whole thing should work from the position of having to justify obstructions. These particular restrictions would not seem necessary unless, again, it was presumed that there was something intrinsically objectionable about the idea of payment in itself. Proposals such as these constitute progress of a kind, but still contain all kinds of restrictions that would not have been applied if there had not been such contrary feeling in the first place. In their very caution they serve, in some ways, to entrench that feeling.

There is no point, in contexts like these, in speculating about motives. Apart from anything else, people can have bad motives while putting forward good arguments, and vice versa. The only way to make progress in a serious moral enquiry is to keep closely to fundamental principles of good reasoning. This is not at all easy. It has to be learned, and to people who engage in it seriously it seems a never-ending quest—although one during which clear progress is often made. But it is absolutely essential for moral seriousness of the deep kind.

The matter of distinguishing between *principles* whose purpose is to *constrain* subsequent policy options, and policies themselves, is crucial to the analysis of most complex questions in practical ethics. Its importance will immediately appear again in the next chapter, about procurement from the dead.

4

PROCUREMENT FROM THE DEAD

Traditions of death

Quite apart from any question of payment, the business of cutting into a living body and extracting healthy organs from it is not something anyone regards as intrinsically desirable. It is true that transplanted organs tend to do better when they come from living donors—the fresher the organ, the better it is likely to fare in its new home—and in some places most kidney transplants come from living donors. But to the extent that we could find less drastic ways of achieving comparably good ends we would on the whole prefer to take them. Unless they have religious commitments that forbid it, most people are likely to accept that as far as possible it is better to use the organs of the dead—which will anyway soon decay, or burn, or be eaten by vultures—than cut into the living. If we can intercept the processes of decay and destruction by removing parts that are no longer of any use to their deceased owner, and give them to others who can get immense benefits from them, that sounds at least on the face of it like an unequivocally good thing.

This obvious fact has led several moral philosophers to say, robustly, that we should use all viable organs of the dead as a matter of routine. The state, on behalf of all of us, should lay claim to whatever parts of dead bodies can be of use to the living, and pass them to transplanters and researchers. It would be a kind of inheritance tax: the state would take parts of the body just as its takes parts of the estate, with the great advantage of not depriving the heirs of anything they would be likely to want for themselves.

Once again, however, the procurement of organs runs up against the problem that transplantation came into a world that had not anticipated it. Humanity has been disposing of its dead for as long as it has existed—ritual disposal of the dead might even be counted as marking the beginning of the species—and the evidence shows not only that all societies have had very specific ways of going about it, but also that it has always mattered a great deal to the people involved. Individuals during their lives have often diverted large proportions of their resources into the preparation of their tombs and funerals, from the ones who could commandeer armies of slaves to construct pyramids and terracotta armies, to the people—within living memory—who anxiously set aside parts of small incomes to avoid the indignity of a pauper's funeral. Conversely, the same concerns have always been used the other way round: threats of what might happen after death have been used to keep the living in order. The Church refused Christian burial to suicides (Ophelia could not be given full Christian burial because 'her death was doubtful'), and the severity of capital punishment could be increased by degrading treatment of the body. The 1720 Murder Act in the UK, for instance, actually specified that executed murderers should not be buried at all—just left hanging in chains to rot—and also allowed for their being condemned to dissection as well as execution.

Demonstration of respect for the dead has also always been a matter of great importance to the honour of surviving families or compatriots. We know from ancient history and legend about the importance of proper funerals, and even now proper disposal of their dead is of great importance to most people. Poor families in many parts of the world are driven into debt, or more deeply into debt, by the social need to provide what they regard as suitable funerals. And, conversely, hostility to the living has often been expressed by contemptuous treatment of their dead: Hector dragged round the walls of Troy and American soldiers through the streets of Mogadishu, desecration of Jewish graves by neo-Nazis, and the bodies of vivisectionists exhumed by animal rights protestors.

Many of these traditions and attitudes were at least originally underpinned by beliefs about what would happen after death. When rulers were buried with possessions and servants it was presumably because they expected to need them in the next life; people who paid for chantry chapels and masses thought it would lessen their time in purgatory; and I also once heard (but have not been able to confirm) of a North Yorkshire family who were buried standing up so that they could rush more quickly to get to the front on the Day of Judgement. Concerns about the interests of the dead have also been interwoven with fears about the harm that might be done by restless spirits if they were not treated properly. It is to be expected, then, that as beliefs of these kinds recede, there will be more scope for changes in attitudes to the treatment of the dead. Most Christians, the creeds notwithstanding, no longer believe in the literal resurrection of the dead, or at least in the need for the original substantial body to serve as its basis; and that, presumably in connection with increasing pressure on burial space, led to the relatively recent acceptability of cremation in the Christian West. There has also for some time been an increasing rationalist tradition of refusing to regard dead bodies as having any intrinsic value, and of willingness to donate them to science for the good of the living.

But still, even where traditional beliefs do not continue, old habits may. The Victorians who protected their dead against the 'resurrection men', who dug up bodies to sell to anatomists, have been followed by the Alder Hey[1] parents who rounded up for separate funerals the parts of their dead children discovered to have been retained as laboratory specimens, and the people who hunted through the World Trade Centre for body parts and put enormous effort into identifying them, and the tribal peoples who campaign to have their ancestors' remains returned for proper burial by the Western museums that have made them into anthropological displays. And even the most committed advocates of transplantation will admit that although of course they would consent to donating the organs of their spouses or children or parents, they would find it emotionally difficult.

It is hardly surprising, therefore, that procuring parts of the dead for transplant is not the straightforward matter that some hardbitten secularists think it should be. Even where retrieval of organs is not in direct conflict with tradition it is almost bound to involve a deviation from it, and deviations in funerary matters have been conventional expressions of, at best, lack of respect. As a result, the tendency in both law and medical convention has been to provide reassurance that organs will not be taken inappropriately.

Although the rights of the living were well established in law long before transplantation came on the scene, the dead and their families had been in no need of similar protection because nobody else had much interest in bodies. But as bodies became useful to other people it became essential to clarify matters, and those clarifications have mainly taken the form of formalizing the rights individuals and families took it for granted they already had. This process began when bodies first became important for anatomical research and teaching; and now, when just about all body parts have become potentially valuable for one purpose or another, their availability has become subject to increasingly strong public insistence on the need for proper consent. In most places, in medical practice even if not in law, organs will not be retrieved without positive consent from either the deceased individual or the family, or in the face of objection by either. Even in cases where the deceased individual has positively given consent before death by joining the transplant register, and where the law allows automatic retrieval of organs, the medical team will not usually proceed in the face of family opposition.

Against this background, debates about how to get more organs from the deceased go on all the time, but rarely lead to anything very radical. Proposals to change transplant registers from opting in to opting out look significant, and certainly arouse strong feelings, but in practice the outcome makes relatively little difference because nearly all such systems are 'soft' in giving the final say to the relatives. Suggestions may be made such as that medical teams should be compelled to raise the question of transplantation with relatives ('required request'), or that everyone should have to register their preferences one way or other, but this is about as far as suggestions for compulsion go. On the whole what emerges from these deliberations amounts to nothing more thoroughgoing than campaigns for public information and education, supplemented by recruitment and training of transplant coordinators. As already commented, the entire transplant community lives in constant fear of scandal-seeking journalists and public backlash, and most of its members are reluctant to suggest anything more positive.

To people who have already reached the conclusion that dead bodies should be used to help the living rather than left to rot, it probably seems that the main obstruction to getting more cadaveric organs lies in popular conservatism about the appropriate treatment of the dead, and that all we can do is wait for public opinion to catch up. This was my own assumption at the start of this analysis. The way the arguments have turned out, however, suggests a significantly different set of conclusions, and quite different possibilities for increasing organ procurement.

The whole issue of deceased donation has turned out to be much more complicated than it seemed at first, and pulling the disparate elements of the public debate into a coherent account is not easy. There is more to be done, but this is the most systematic account I have been able to manage so far. I hope it catches the essentials.

Opting in and out: a methodological case study

Consider, both as an object lesson in methodology and as a launching pad for the substantial discussion, the debate about whether the policy of organ donation should work by opting in (putting yourself on the donation register) or opting out (putting yourself on a register of non-donors). This question recently arose as a live public issue in the UK because the Prime Minister at the time was anxious to increase the organ donation rate, and asked an already existing Donation Taskforce[2] to look into the matter.

It may be worth saying—just as an illustration of the tribulations of moral reasoning in practice—that my own investigation of deceased donation originally began with an analysis of this question, because it seemed to lend itself ideally to the approach outlined at the beginning of the book. Since people never do or could get round to doing all the things they would like to do, a system that made organs available as a result of inaction looked certain to produce more organs for transplant than one that relied on people's acting on their good intentions. This suggested that the analysis could be set up in the way already described, with a presumption in favour of opting out, and a challenge to opters-in to show how that presumption could be defeated. However, after long efforts to engage with various parts of the public debate, and the generation of reams of detailed argument and dozens of diagrams, I eventually concluded that such a direct approach was hopeless, and the whole lot had to be discarded.

The reasons for this were essentially the ones that now appear at the end of the previous chapter. The problem was that the public debate was about whether to change to a *policy* of opting out, which produced an unsorted mass of ideas about anything that might possibly be relevant under any circumstances: claims about the likelihood of backlashes, the different kinds of way in which families might be involved, whether opters out or opters in would be more likely to register, how much time would have to be allowed for change, how much change would cost, evidence about what had happened in other countries, how we could find out what the dead would have wanted, what recipients thought about the matter, and a hundred other miscellaneous issues.

So, for instance, one of the questions that kept coming up was whether changing to a policy of opting out would actually increase the numbers of organs donated. This is a complicated empirical question. It is no good just comparing countries that have instigated this system with ones that have not, because there might be all kinds of background issues that influenced the overall outcome in different places. Anyway the involvement of families—a problem in its own right—complicated things still further, since nobody seemed willing to attempt a hard opting-out system (where the organs of people who had not opted out would be used without any consultation of the family). As long as families had the power of veto there might be very little difference in practice between the two systems. A change to opting out might even reduce the numbers of organs available by generating an adverse public reaction of some kind, producing droves of opters out indignant about the idea of the state's laying claim to their organs, or afraid of what might happen to them if they could be recognized in advance as potential organ donors. Many people involved in the debate—and the report of the Taskforce—claimed that it was far from certain that a change to opting out would result in any increase in numbers of available organs at all. Since increasing the rate of donation was the whole purpose of the proposed change, it seemed as though this should be the first question to resolve; but it also seemed pretty intractable.

If the problem of opting in and out is to be approached as a systematic enquiry, there is no point in just plunging in and engaging with all the elements in the public debate. The questions first need to be got into a systematic order, because the answers given to the more fundamental questions will determine whether the others need to be addressed at all, and what their relevance is. This is where the material of the final section of the previous chapter comes in. The question about opting in and out is, like so many other questions, one that can be understood either as an all-things-considered question about policy, or as a question about rights that should be accepted as fundamental *constraints* on the details of any acceptable policy. If you think we should accept as a *fundamental principle* that organs should not be used without positive consent, that in itself settles the policy question. The other questions, about cost and timing and backlashes do not even arise. On the other hand, if you do not think there should be such a principle, the question about policy remains open, with the possibility that a system of opting in might still be regarded as the best on other grounds. Obviously the first question to ask is the one of principle.

Once this point has been recognized, it becomes striking that it was nowhere addressed as such in the public debate. But at the same time there were innumerable indications that many people took it for granted that the right not to have organs retrieved without positive consent should be regarded as fundamental.

It was clear, in the first place, that many people believed that this idea was widely and strongly held by others, whether or not they held it themselves. For instance, it is often said that it would be quite impossible to establish an opting-out system in societies without educated populations. That claim implies a belief that the public would not accept the use of bodies unless everyone could reasonably be presumed to understand the situation, so that failure to opt out could be treated as amounting to positive consent. It is also shown in the general fear that there might be a public backlash if opting out were introduced, implying that people could be expected to feel resentment at being deprived of something they already regarded as a right. It also seems indicated by the extreme difficulty of getting hard opting-out systems established—in which organs can, in theory, be retrieved without consultation of the family of the deceased. There is clearly a deep feeling that *someone* should give positive consent for organ retrieval. The same idea also appears in the indignation many people express at describing opting-out systems as ones of 'presumed consent'. There is no reason why this should not be a legally acceptable description of a policy, but if you think there should be a fundamental entitlement to positive consent, you may well regard this description as sleight of hand.

There is also direct evidence that many people do themselves believe that positive consent should be required for organ donation as a matter of principle, even though it is rarely stated in quite those terms, because it can be inferred from the arguments they present in favour of keeping a policy of opting in. For instance, in one broadcast discussion a participant gave as an objection to opting out that it would allow for the possibility that some isolated, ignorant person could have their organs used against their real wishes. The fact that this was treated as manifestly appalling, even though other lives would be saved and the person concerned would never know anything about it, shows that the speaker was regarding this as a fundamental right, overriding any calculation of harms and benefits.

The same assumption is also indicated in less obvious ways. For instance, the report of the UK Taskforce says a great deal about how essential it would be, if the current policy were to be changed to one of opting out, to have a long lead-in time during which it could be made certain that everyone knew what the situation was. There was no mention at all of the lives that would be lost while we took such care to make sure that all organs used were from positively willing donors. This argument *presupposes* that the default right is the strong one—a need for positive consent—and that any change would need safeguards so strong as to guarantee pretty well the same thing. Elsewhere in the same document, one of the concerns expressed was about the difficulty of ensuring that people who opted out could do so without anyone knowing, so that they did not run the risk of public disapprobation. This is also an indication, though an interestingly subtle one, that the people who brought this matter up regarded the right to give positive consent as fundamental (or at least, were concerned about a public who thought it so). If we have a right to something, we do not normally regard ourselves as having to give justifications when we make use of that right. Most of us do not feel a perpetual need to justify keeping other people out of our house or holding on to our property, and we are regarded as—and probably feel—positively generous to the extent that we waive such rights in the interests of others. That is the situation with organ donation in an opting-in system. But if the default is in the other direction, and we have to take positive action to prevent donation, not donating looks actively mean. The concern that people should be able to opt out in privacy therefore amounts to a presupposition in favour of a strong right not to donate (a right that does not make you look mean if you do not join the donation register), and that if we decide to weaken that right by having an opting-out system, we should try to make sure that as many as possible of its old accoutrements—not having to appear in public as mean—are still around. So the first question to be resolved seems to be whether we should accept as a fundamental principle that organs are not used unless there is positive consent.

But in fact there is an even more fundamental matter to sort out, which is exactly what the fundamental rights being demanded are supposed to be. This may sound obvious, but there are several real puzzles here. The most conspicuous of these concerns the relationship of deceased individuals and their surviving families. If both individuals and the families are supposed to have rights over dead bodies, how are these supposed to connect with each other? In particular, whose should trump whose in cases of conflict? In practice, at the moment, it seems to be the case that consent from either quarter is necessary for donation, but also that refusal from either quarter is sufficient to prevent it. Is that what is intended? We need to be clear about what any proposal is before we can begin the process of assessing it. And it turns out that when an attempt is made to clarify the issue of which rights should belong to each of the two groups, other problems quickly arise about how to understand the nature of the relevant rights.

The public debate is no use as a guide. The various elements can be brought in as they seem relevant, but when the analysis is properly structured many of them may turn out to be of no importance. The first problem to sort out is this matter of rights, and in particular how the rights of individuals and families connect.

Individual rights

Many people seem to take it for granted that nobody should take our organs without positive consent, but it is interesting to consider exactly why. A problem arises here comparable to one discussed earlier (Ch. 3, p. 123) in the context of organ selling. When organ selling first came to light the condemnation was direct and immediate, but this could not have been a response learned from other people's reactions and social pressure, because the phenomenon was so new. Nor could it be a response either to selling or to taking organs from a living body, since neither of these was on its own regarded as objectionable. This raised the interesting question of why the combination of the two should seem so self-evidently wrong. It must have seemed, intuitively, to belong to some already recognizable, objectionable, category. The same question arises here. When the possibility of cadaveric transplants became known, many people made an equally immediate presumption that organ retrieval should not happen without positive consent. This suggests that it must immediately have been recognized, intuitively, as coming into some existing category of rights. But which category, exactly? If we are to get to the root of the question of rights over dead bodies, it seems important to try to understand what precisely seemed immediately wrong about the unauthorized removal of organs.

The most obvious possibility lies in a contravention of some accepted, established rights of the dead. But what are the traditional rights of the dead over their bodies? When you try to pin them down, there seem to have been remarkably few. You have the right to have your property disposed of according to a properly formulated will, and you could in that way make provision for funerals and tombs and monuments, but otherwise you had no formal control over what happened to you. Your family might feel a strong personal duty to fulfil your known wishes, and would certainly feel that they had social as well as personal obligations to dispose of your body respectfully. But you yourself had no legal rights to having anything positive done by other people. Traditionally you never even had the right to what would be regarded as a decent burial—though in present-day welfare states you presumably have. There have been all kinds of requirements concerned with public health and decency about the disposal of bodies, but those are not rights of the disposed-of individual. In fact such requirements have always constituted constraints on what individuals might choose to have done—as in the case of people who would like to be buried in unsanctioned places, or the man who was not allowed to have his body made into food for the Battersea Dogs' Home.

Furthermore, none of these limited rights concern what will happen to you by default unless you give positive consent for something else. In all these cases you would have to make positive efforts to set the arrangements up, either by making provisions in your will, or by making it clear to your family what you hoped would happen. And to the extent that these things are rights at all (you might say that you had a conventional right to expect your family to go along with your wishes, even if not a legal one) they are *positive* rights, in the sense that they impose positive obligations on particular other people to do particular things for you. In both respects these rights of the dead are quite unlike the implied right not to have your body parts used for transplants. The right not to be used in the absence of consent is in its essence not one you need to activate: the default is that you will not be used. Nor is this right one that involves the imposition of positive duties on others. It is a *negative* right, which requires *everyone* to *refrain* from doing something to you. So it is hard to see anything in the traditional rights of the dead from which a right of this kind could be naturally inferred.

This makes it look as though the default right required is something like an extension of the rights of the living: something equivalent to the right not to be killed or assaulted or kidnapped. These are rights we all have against everyone, meaning that everyone has a negative duty not to kill or assault or kidnap us, or even touch us inappropriately without our consent. These are also rights that we have by default, not ones that we have to invoke: nobody thinks we are open to assault or murder unless we opt out of them. This too seems in line with the idea that we should have to give positive consent for organ donation. We should in some way be regarded as sacrosanct even after we are dead, just as we are when alive, and not interfered with without our consent.

However, although this idea is intuitively plausible, it immediately runs into problems. The dead cannot possibly have rights that take anything like the form of these fundamental rights of the living. The whole point of surrounding us, in life, with a circle of rights that other people cannot infringe without consent is to make certain things dependent on our will, and set them beyond the scope of what can be done to us by others. But when we are dead we can do *nothing* for ourselves. Everything has to be done to us, and this must, by default, be without our consent. Bodies cannot just be left lying around because their deceased owner has not given advance permission for disposal; and it would be impossible, anyway, to anticipate everything that might need to be done and give consent for it. There is also no sign that anyone has ever suggested rights of this form. Very few people now, probably, have much idea of what is going to happen to them when they die, and most of us may well not want to know. Once again, we may make specific requests, but otherwise the default procedures just go ahead without any consultation or advance consent at all.

So the default situation with the dead has never been, and never could be, that bodies should be left untouched except in ways for which specific consent had been given. If there is to be a negative right of some kind—a right not to have certain things done after death unless you give positive consent—it cannot just be the generalized not-touching, not-interfering rights recognized for the living. This means that this right, whatever it is, needs to be specified. We need to be clear about *which* things count as infringements of some default right, under which taking organs for transplant would automatically be recognized as falling. And again, since we have such an intuitive and strong feeling about this question, it looks as though it should be something pretty well established.

Still, it is still hard to see what this might be. There might in principle be conventions about things that could not be done in the way of disposal without advance consent, but there do not seem in fact to be any established rights of this kind. There are certainly none so well established that everyone's intuition would immediately pick them up. As already mentioned, there are constraints of public propriety, but nothing that comes into the category of rights of the deceased.

A more plausible idea, in this context, is that there might be a default presumption that people should be disposed of in one piece: an understood right to be burnt or buried whole unless you positively gave consent for anything else. But even though it is more plausible, it again does not seem to correspond with any established convention. People have sometimes kept amputated limbs specifically to be buried with them, and there may be some cultures where it is regarded as necessary for bodies to be intact; but that is not the case in many of the cultures where people intuitively think it wrong to take organs without consent. For instance, there never seems to have been any general expectation that organs and tissues excised during surgical operations should be preserved for later burial—even in cases where the patient may have died during or immediately after the operation. These body parts have traditionally been disposed of as a matter of routine, and if you positively wanted to keep them for some reason, you needed to make a specific request. There is also the routine draining of blood for embalming, which seems to be generally accepted, and there is a long tradition of burying hearts in different places from the rest of the body. It was also common to take bits and pieces of saints to different places as relics, even when the resurrection of the dead 'in this flesh' was the literal expectation. There never seems to have been any general expectation of wholeness in disposal.

However, other relatively recent developments suggest a different explanation of what really underlies these feelings. It was for a long time taken for granted that tissues and organs removed in the course of surgery would simply be disposed of at the time, without any requirement that they should be kept for eventual disposal with the rest of their owner, or even that their disposal required positive consent. The trouble started when it was realized that they were not being disposed of, but being kept for other purposes: as specimens for research and teaching, or, in particular, for the money-making activities of pharmaceutical companies. In these cases the concern was obviously not the fate of the body parts as such, but the fact that someone else was *making use of you* without your consent. It is difficult to see what else could be the real issue underlying anxiety about the unauthorized use of organs for transplant, especially in the case of bodies destined for cremation. It seems to be not the removal of the organs as such, or their separation from the original body, but their being used—without positive authorization—as a means to someone else's ends. In other words, the insistence on consent seems to have far less to do with traditions about the treatment of bodies, which the long history of concern for treatment of the dead might suggest, than with something akin to the ownership of property.

There are many reasons for thinking this is likely to be true. For instance, the Alder Hey parents who collected the scattered parts of their children and gave them separate funerals said that they had let down their children by not burying them whole. But they also complained that the organs had been retained *without consent*—and consent would not have been relevant if wholeness had been the issue.[3] We might also consider what would happen if funeral directors were discovered to have sold the blood drained from dead bodies to research laboratories or fertilizer manufacturers, rather than just disposing of it. Or you might consider the difference between anticipating that your own heart might be removed without your consent, for experiments or transplantation, and it being removed by admirers who wanted to put it in a shrine. That is an interesting question (and the response may well differ between people) but it suggests a possible difference of attitude towards activities still devoted to you, in some way, and ones where you are treated as a means to someone else's ends. The essence of all these matters seems to be not so much *what* is done to your body, as *why* it is done. If it is done with you and your interests—including your posthumous interests—in mind, that is fine; if you are being made a means to someone else's ends, consent is required.

If this is right, there are slightly different ways in which this attitude could be interpreted. One is as an objection to being used *merely as a means*—which we think is wrong when people are alive. The other is a matter of property: people taking what is *yours* for their own purposes, without your positive agreement. In practice, structurally, these ideas come out as much the same. So what I want to suggest here is that the root of the feeling that positive consent is needed for posthumous organ donation can best be understood as a variation of our feelings about property rights. For instance, if undertakers sold the drained blood of dead people without consent, that would seem wrong in much the same way as if they stole the wedding rings of people about to be cremated.

It has already been suggested, in the context of organ selling, that as transplantation became established people intuitively and automatically regarded their organs as *theirs* in much the same way as any other property. This attitude also seems to be officially endorsed at least to the extent that it keeps being stressed that organ donation, either before or after the death of the donor, is a matter of making a *gift*. It is something that no one has any right to expect, but whose offering would show great generosity on the part of the owner. But the idea that usable body parts are thought of as essentially property is suggested by other evidence as well. For instance, here are two of the reactions of journalists during the UK's debate, objecting vociferously to any idea of a switch to opting out:

> The idea lets in an evil and dangerous political principle—the assumption that the state owns our bodies. Brown [the Prime Minister] and Labour governments before him have tried to

nationalise our private lives; now he wants to nationalise our private parts.[4]

Gordon Brown has appropriated just about everything we own, so it is no surprise that he is now trying to nationalise our bodies, by introducing a law of 'presumed consent' for organ donations, unless people specifically opt out...Presumed consent would be the ultimate victory of the New Labour totalitarians: the acknowledgement that they own us down to the last sinew and tissue. It must be rejected.[5]

Both of these imply that the issue is essentially a matter of ownership and property. Another interesting indication of the same idea is that if the deceased owner of the organs has said nothing about what is to happen to them, the right to make the decision routinely passes to the surviving family. This is more or less the case with other property in the case of intestacy. I shall say more about this in the next section.

The idea that our organs are essentially our property, which other people have no right to take for their own purposes without consent, seems to me the most plausible interpretation of what underlies many of the ways these matters are thought of, discussed, and reacted to. No doubt at the level of psychology there are many other relevant issues, such as simple squeamishness, and unwillingness to think about what happens after death, as well traditional expectations about how bodies should be treated. But the property issue looks like a significant element, and worth taking seriously.

I had presumed before starting this enquiry that what underlay individuals' resistance to donate their organs was a simple concern about what would happen to the body itself after death. Like many other people who are keen to make the best possible use of dead bodies for the good of the living, I regarded this resistance as essentially a superstitious residue of pre-scientific beliefs, out of which people needed to be persuaded. This seems to underlie the familiar idea that what is needed to increase donation is public education: that if we can persuade individuals that what happens to their body after death makes no difference to them personally, they will cheerfully agree to donation. If the rights people demand are a relic of superstition, our policy, in a democracy, should be to change their minds through education.

But if the real underlying concern is something more like ideas of property rights, that seems to me to cast a different and rather surprising light on the matter. It is not difficult to understand why people want to keep their own property, rather than give it away; but there is, of course, one respect in which organs are quite unlike other property. Your organs cannot be of any use to you after you are dead. This seems to imply that if you want the right not to have your organs used without your positive consent, or even the weaker right to be able to prevent their use, what you are in effect demanding is the right to *waste* them. If the issue of organ donation is essentially one of property rather than treatment of bodies, giving people the right not to have their organs used is to give them the right to be dogs in mangers: to prevent other people from getting what they can no longer use themselves.

When the matter is put like this, it probably sounds appalling that people should have—or indeed want—any rights at all over the use of their bodies when they are dead. It may seem to lead directly to the moral conclusion that the state should indeed requisition all dead bodies; or, at the very least, that you should have to go to the trouble of deliberately opting out of having your body used. This is, of course, what many people already think.

But although I personally agree that these are the policies we should be aiming for, I also suspect that the matter is more complex than it looks. It seems likely that dog-in-a-mangery, in some form, is likely to be pretty deep in human nature. Although we know that natural selection can produce considerable altruism, we also know that what succeeds in the evolutionary competition is not just how well you yourself do, but how well you do *in comparison with others*, or how well your group does in comparison with other groups. Evolutionary success must often involve a disposition to deprive rivals of what might enhance their success. And I wonder—another speculation that is worth raising, even though I have not yet had time to explore it much—whether the deep concern of people who want to prevent the use of their dead bodies by others is not so much about the right to *prevent* their use, as to have *control* over their use—or at least, not to give unknown others control of their use. In other words, the depth of the feeling that organ donation should not happen without our positive consent may lie less in a wish to *prevent* the use of organs than to *control* it. At present, it is widely taken for granted that organs from the dead should become public goods, to be allocated impartially, on the basis of need.

In other words, the difference in people's attitudes to organ donation may be connected with wider attitudes to ideas about the state, private property, and the public good. This would be an interesting question for empirical research, and I would predict some correlation between attitudes to public control of organs and attitudes to public and private property in general. In the meantime, if this is on the right lines, it may explain why there is far more disagreement about rights over bodies when they are dead than there is about our rights over our bodies when we are alive, and also about how to increase organ procurement in a liberal society.

I shall raise this matter again below, in the two sections on impartiality of distribution (pp. 175 and 188). First, however, there is the question of how the fundamental rights of individuals—whatever anyone thinking through the problems decides those should be—should connect with those of the surviving family.

Families

If all this is on the right lines, it suggests once again that the newness, in historical terms, of the ability to pass body parts from one person to another, is the reason why people's strong intuitions about the matter of donation are so confused and difficult to deal with.

There are two distinct aspects to dealing with death, which have traditionally been quite separate. One is disposal of the body, along with funeral rites and memorials, which have mattered a great deal both to individuals in anticipation of death and to families and other groups afterwards. The other is the disposal of property. Until very recently these two elements had nothing to do with each other, and the matter of disposal could be regarded as self-contained. Now, if the foregoing arguments are on the right track, the matter of donation is one that people seem to class intuitively with property issues and bequests. This feeling is not yet explicit or complete, partly because we still seem resistant to regarding body parts as commodities, and in law bodies can still not be treated as property. But it must also partly be because, as a matter of fact, organ donation has mixed up categories that were previously kept entirely distinct. The matter of ensuring the correct disposal of property has always been separate from the matter of disposal of the body, and to a large extent in different hands. Because organ retrieval must inevitably be dealt with as part of the physical aspects of death, the matter of donation has become in effect part of the process of disposal rather than of bequests. This is where the confusions about family involvement arise.

It is easy to see why the matter of consent to donation has been in the hands of families. Families have always been responsible for disposal of bodies, not because anyone had demanded this as a right, but because bodies had to be disposed of, and the person 'in lawful possession' of the body had a duty to see that this was appropriately done. For most of history most people died at home, with their family as the obvious lawful possessors of the body, and the family would also be concerned to dispose of the dead with proper respect.

When hospitals eventually became places of medical expertise—as opposed to the charitable refuges for the poor that they had been for most of history—people began to die there, not by design, but because that became the best place to go for help as they became increasingly ill. But hospitals automatically restored lawful possession to the family, who took it for granted that disposal was their responsibility and would not normally consider the social disgrace of handing the body over to the parish, or whatever public organization was responsible for unclaimed bodies. So it is not surprising that both families and clinicians take it for granted that families are responsible for what happens after death, or that, whatever the law says, the professionals involved hesitate to interfere with the process of disposal unless they have the family's consent.

Quite apart from legal and formal traditions, there is also the matter of care of the dying, with which clinicians and families are usually both involved. The patients who are most likely to be appropriate donors are ones in intensive care, where the medical team will have been doing everything possible to save the life of the patient, and usually interacting all the time with a distraught family. Unless the family itself anticipates and raises the issue, there is nowhere in all this that a request for organ donation naturally comes. The business of making the request is gratingly inappropriate in the situation, from both sides' points of view, and it is not surprising if clinicians cannot bring themselves to do it. (It is the recognition of this difficulty that leads to proposals such as 'required request'.) Nor is it surprising that, even when they are asked, the family often refuses. Like the clinicians, they want to concentrate all their care and attention on the dying person; and when death eventually happens, families usually do not feel a sudden end to their duty of care. It is often difficult to take on board the reality of death, especially of the relatively young person whose death is sudden. A family, whose duty is by all tradition towards the care of the dying and dead, may not happily agree to something that may seem like allowing an additional trauma—a further assault. 'He's suffered enough.'

Essentially, the problem is that the issue of deceased donation arises in a context where, for reasons that long predated any question of transplantation, matters were automatically in the hands of the relatives. This means that in practice donation has come to be classified as part of the disposal issues: a matter to be dealt with by bereavement counselling, rather than some equivalent of probate, which covers property and bequests. The important question for public policy is whether we should complete the transition, and formally recognize the issue of organ donation as an aspect of bequests. This does seem to be how most individuals regard it when they opt into the transplant register.

If this is the right way to look at the matter, it is clear by all our normal standards that the family should not be able to override the individual's properly stated wishes. The family has no power at all to override a will.* If you leave all your money to the cats' home, the cats get it, quite irrespective of what your family thinks about the matter; and my guess is that most people, if asked directly, would say that the expressed wishes of the deceased should not be overruled by the family.

Of course, there is also the matter of family distress to consider—and it will be pointed out that since families so often do refuse donation, there must be distress involved. But, quite apart from the fact that relatives can be as distressed as they like about the cats without its making any difference, there is an important question here about the real roots of any distress. If the problem for the relatives is their continued feeling of care, it is at least possible—I would say plausible—that the distress may lie less in the procurement itself than in the idea of giving permission for it. The very fact of families' being asked for consent implies that the responsibility is theirs, and as their traditional duty was to arrange respectful disposal this may seem like a serious intrusion on their

* A court may sometimes do this on behalf of a family in cases where it judges there is a specific entitlement.

responsibilities. But if it were taken for granted that the wishes of the deceased would be implemented automatically—as in the case of wills, or coroners' autopsies—and that everything went ahead routinely behind the scenes, it is not obvious that families would suffer any more than they now do from legally required post mortems, or, indeed, from what goes on in the ordinary handling of bodies by undertakers. If families still personally prepared the bodies of the dead it would be different, but the relatives of potential donors are not often in that position. Most people now probably prefer not to think about what goes on behind the scenes: these things are just accepted as other people's responsibility. If the removal of organs for transplants were similarly taken for granted—classified as bequests—the distress might simply go. Of course, there is enormous variation in family traditions between different cultures, but a change of this kind in the law would not affect that—because people with such traditions could specify that their families should make the decision.

It should also be added that such a separation would make things much easier, and more congenial, for clinical teams responsible for the care of dying patients. There would be no need to interrupt the care of the family with requests for organ donation, since the matter would have been settled—and recorded on readily available registers—in advance. There would also be no need for any of the difficulties encountered in many places in trying to decide exactly at which point in the dying process to raise the subject with families. At the moment many clinicians (depending on jurisdiction) face the tricky problem that if families are asked for consent to donation too soon—before they have given up hope—they may refuse, but if the matter is left until later, when they are more likely to consent, it will be too late to keep the organs in the best possible state. If donation were settled in advance, matters of preservation and retrieval could be dealt with automatically, by recognized, established protocols.

There would still be many logistical problems, of course; the physical aspects of the two elements, death and donation, cannot be separated as simply as the legalities might be. There would be a good deal to work out about how best to manage organ preservation and retrieval without disturbing the relatives more than absolutely necessary. But if the matter were clarified—if the law made it clear that the two issues were quite distinct as a matter of procedure even though it was impossible to separate them entirely in practice—people who already understand the mechanics and psychology of both transplantation and death could put their minds to getting the two as technically separated and as smoothly managed as possible.

All this, of course, would apply only to people who had actually specified their wishes in some formally approved way. That would still leave the people who had not specified their wishes. Should relatives make the decision here? That would probably seem the most natural default, since there is some kind of natural way in which property rights in the body seem to belong to the family. If people die intestate, the family usually inherits by default. So, in the case of the deceased whose wishes were undeclared, it would be quite in line with much of our normal thinking to say that the family should take over the role of inheritor.

What this implies, given how few people get round to opting in, is that such an arrangement would leave matters in many ways similar to the present situation. In practice the families would still have to be asked in most cases. If we wanted to make a significant difference to the way things are currently done, we would probably have to make more radical changes to present arrangements.

This raises the quite different subject matter of the next two sections.

Impartiality of distribution 1: directed donation

This chapter on procurement from the dead, like the earlier one on procurement from the living, began with a discussion of impediments to procurement already entrenched in tradition before the possibility of transplants arose. In the case of the dead, most of these were merely traditions rather than legally established rights, but people feel strongly about them and most seem to want something of the kind entrenched in law.

However, as in the case of living donation, not all the obstacles to organ procurement are of this traditional kind, deep in people's feelings about themselves and their bodies. Others involve rules that actually *go against* the uses that individuals might like to make of the new technological possibilities. Organ selling, in particular, was not something into which people had to be persuaded against their natural inclinations. The exchange of organs for money was instigated by the people involved themselves, who clearly presumed that organs already recognized as theirs to give must also be theirs to sell. Organ selling was made illegal, and its implementation declared contrary to professional standards, by people who had no direct interest in the matter, and in spite of its inevitably reducing the legitimate organ supply.

The next topic in the area of deceased donation is another of this same general kind. Just as people might reasonably presume, when organs became transferable, that they were entitled to sell them, so people who are asked to donate their organs after their death might reasonably presume that, as in the case of other bequests, they should be allowed to specify where their donations went. It is constantly emphasized to prospective donors that if they do allow donation this will be a generous gift: something that nobody has any right to expect, but whose giving would be an act of wonderful altruism. Our normal presumption about gifts and bequests, however, is that it is up to the donor to decide not only whether they are given or not, but also who is going to get them.

In the case of living donation it is more or less required that you say whom your organ is going to. So-called Samaritan donation, although increasingly accepted, is still widely regarded with suspicion. But with deceased organ donation this is generally not the case: it is widely insisted that deceased organ donation must be absolutely undirected. For instance, when it turned out a few years ago that some people in the UK had agreed to donate the organs of a deceased relative as long as they could make conditions about acceptable recipients, and the transplant team had agreed, the reaction of the establishment was nearly as immediate and decisive as in the case of the discovery of organ selling. Even though there had been beforehand no official prohibition of such conditional donation, the transplant team involved was treated as though it should have known that this was totally unacceptable in principle. The government (as usual) convened an advisory group which issued a report,[6] and explicit policy was introduced to say that only organs offered unconditionally could be accepted. It is now widely, if not

universally, held that deceased organs must be donated unconditionally, to be allocated impartially to whoever is at the top of the
list.[7]

However, the very fact that people have tried to make conditions
shows that at least some do care not just about whether their organs
are used, but also about who gets them. This is, of course, strongly
in line with the speculations at the end of the section before last,
and suggests that at least some part of the resistance to organ donation may be the feeling that you would be handing parts of yourself
over to goodness knows whom. Perhaps the recipients might be
people whose life you would rather not save, or at least people to
whom you would give a low priority. If when you die you are taken
straight to the funeral establishment, and just disposed of, at least
you know that nothing of you is going for purposes of which you
might disapprove.

The idea that the requirement of unconditionality might be a
significant obstacle to donation seems to be felt by many people
who work with racial minorities. Racial and cultural minorities
are underrepresented as donors, and this is no doubt partly because of cultural traditions. But marginal groups may well also
have a general distrust of the establishment, and one of the elements of the suspicion may be that their group is likely to be
discriminated against in distribution. They may think that any
organ they donated would probably be used by the dominant
group for its own benefit. More generally (this is just anecdote,
but plausible enough) individuals discussing their attitude to donation often express concern about who might get their organs,
and say they would be willing to donate to some people, but not
others. Organizations such as the UK National Health Service

may be committed to the view that you do not enquire into the moral character or social worth of patients when deciding whom to treat, but individuals rarely feel like that when they are making gifts.

We have no idea how much effect the principle of unconditionality has on supply, since if people know conditions cannot be imposed they will not bother to try. They may just refuse donation. Presumably this is something that would vary with prevailing attitudes in different societies. If we wanted to find which kinds of arrangement would maximize donation we would need to experiment with different systems, allowing different kinds of choice—and, as in the case of organ selling, the very fact that directed donation is not allowed means that we have far too little relevant evidence. However, the fact that some people have tried to impose conditions is significant, and if the policy of insisting that all donations must be unconditional has any effect at all on supply, it must be to diminish it.

Once again, the prohibition of directed donation is not an all-things-considered conclusion reached after a good deal of social experiment. It might in principle be reached that way, but there has been no such experiment. This is another case of a principle that was treated from the outset as a *constraint* on what was allowable. The question is whether any such principle can be justified.

So, given that we also have other presumptions against insisting on unconditionality—our usual attitudes to gifts and bequests— we have the usual problem about how to complete an argument whose starting premises seem to support the opposite conclusion.

The argument needed is something on these lines:

There is a presumption against any policy that may reduce the supply of organs.

Excluding all forms of directed or conditional donation will, if it has any effect on the donation rate, reduce it—perhaps considerably.

Normally, when we give, we say who gets the gift.

This is true even (or especially) in the case of living organ donation.

But...

Therefore we should not allow any form of directed or conditional deceased donation.

Once again, we seem to need a pretty decisive '*But...*' premise. There are various candidates in the field.

One common claim is that directed donation would be unfair because it would involve queue jumping. If someone says that their organs are to go to a window cleaner, that means that a window cleaner low down the waiting list gets pushed to the top. However, it would be a mistake to describe that as queue jumping. If a fellow window cleaner came and offered a living donation, that would obviously not be queue jumping; it would be taking the person out of the queue, by making available something other than what was being queued for—as if you offered a friend in a bus queue a lift in your car. Similarly, a person who makes a directed donation that would otherwise not have been made takes the person who benefits out of the general queue—and since the people ahead in the queue are unaffected, and the ones behind get the advantage of moving forward, nobody has any such ground for complaint.

More generally, queue jumping is something that can take place only against the background of a rule or convention that determines the order of access to some benefit. If an English person, who is used to queuing for buses, goes abroad and finds stampedes at bus stops, it would be nonsense to complain about queue jumping in the local population: the appropriate complaint would be that there was no queuing convention at all. Similarly, if we are asking what the principle of distribution of deceased organs should be, the fact, if it is one, that something would constitute queue jumping against the background of present standards is quite irrelevant to the question of whether those standards should be changed—which is the question here.

Another common objection is that directed or conditional donation allows for racist specifications. This was the complaint in the case that brought the matter of directed donation to public attention in the UK: the relatives of the deceased—who lived in an area of high immigration—agreed to donation as long as the organs went to a white recipient. The transplant team gave the necessary assurances, saying afterwards that a white patient had anyway been at the top of the waiting list and would have been the recipient irrespective of the condition. Nevertheless there was outrage, and when the reporting group presented their defence of disallowing directed donation it gave the possibility of racism as its first reason. The objection raised most commonly in general discussion is also that allowing directed donation would allow for racism.

There is a great deal that might be said about this matter. Racism itself is a much more complex issue than is often allowed by the rhetoric of the way the term is used. If we take it that the word is conventionally applied only to what is morally bad, then it is not at all clear where racism begins and a commendable concern with your own family and friends and social group ends. Would it be racist if a member of some immigrant minority specified a preference for donation to someone within that group? Would it be objectionable if a Jew would prefer to donate to a Jew, or a Muslim to a Muslim? It is very difficult to decide when individual rights should be curtailed in the interests of preventing discrimination. There is also the question, once again, of why there should be arbitrary constraints in the context of organs that do not exist for other gifts and bequests. You can leave money to any individual or cause you like, unless the cause is illegal in itself. Huge amounts of money are given or left to religious groups, ethnically linked charities and community centres, and political parties of all persuasions. If this is not outlawed, it is not clear why similarly directed donation of organs should be unacceptable in principle.

But anyway, quite apart from such details, there is no point in going further (or perhaps even that far) into that particular issue, because it is not relevant to the question of whether directed or conditional donation *in general* should be prohibited. The question here is not about what arrangements for cadaveric donation would be best all things considered, but, once again, whether an objection to any kinds of condition or expression of preference should be a *fundamental* principle, to be accepted as a constraint from the outset of policy debates. An objection to one kind of condition that might be made is not an argument against allowing *any* kind of condition. As before, if some policy is presumptively good—in getting more organs—but is open to abuses of various kinds—as with organ selling—anyone whose objection is seriously about the danger of abuses should be doing what they can to work out ways of avoiding the harm, if possible, while still allowing the good. As it happened, the working group that wrote the UK report thought that the case that prompted the fuss probably contravened the Race Relations Act. If so, the Act itself was enough to prevent anything objectionable in its terms, without there being any need to say that all conditional donation, of any kind, should be refused.

If conditional or directed donation is to be ruled out entirely, from the start—as opposed to being a possible conclusion of a complex enquiry—we need a general principle that would be strong enough to support the conclusion directly. And, in fact, the consultation group did offer one, specifically described in those terms: 'the fundamental principle that organs are donated altruistically and should go to patients in the greatest need'.[8] Once again this may seem to strike the right rhetorical notes, but there are immediate problems.

One of them is about the idea of greatest need in itself, and how the list of criteria for establishing priority is in fact put together. Although this book is about procurement rather than distribution, the matter is perhaps worth a passing comment. It is true that there are waiting lists and publicly formulated criteria for establishing them, but it is misleading to describe them as if some objective standard of need provided the basis of the ordering. In the first place, need is not the only criterion used. Apart from such obvious issues as tissue matching, there are various matters of 'equity' taken into account: length of time on the waiting list, trying to get the probability of getting an organ equal between different groups, and so on. These have nothing to do with need, and may be highly controversial. But even if need were the only issue, any appearance that this is a clear criterion dissolves as soon as any attempt is made to pin it down. If three people are about to die for want of a liver, one of whom is in his sixties and involved in crucial research that will not continue without him, one of whom is a single mother with four dependent children, and one of whom is young and not particularly promising, but with more life ahead of him, whose need is greatest? Or if two people need some organ, one of whom is severely ill and will die soon, but for whom the operation has a low chance of success, and another who is likely to get many years of life from it, but is in less immediate danger of death? There simply is no obvious answer to such questions as these. Impartial allocation principles could take indefinitely many forms, all open to debate, so it is at best misleading to describe the people at the top of the currently constituted list as 'in greatest need'. In fact, many of the people who have no chance of getting on to the list at all may be in what many people would intuitively count as the greatest need, because they are in particularly bad states of health. This is not, I should emphasize, intended as a criticism of any particular set of criteria for ordering. My point is only that the matter is far from clear and simple, and there could be many plausible sets of criteria for constructing a waiting list.

For now at least, however, set that matter aside and consider the principle as it stands. It is not entirely clear how to interpret it—whether the 'and' is intended as linking two separate principles or presenting one as an interpretation of the other. If the reference is to just one 'fundamental principle', it looks as though its implication is not only that altruism is required, but also that altruism consists in willingness to give 'to patients in the greatest need'. This is also suggested by the wider context, since there would otherwise have been no need to mention altruism in the context of unconditional donation: in the general sense of acting in some-one else's interests rather than your own, which is what altruism is, all deceased organ donation is altruistic.

First, as was argued in the organ-selling context, the idea that the only acceptable way to get some resource is through altruism is an extraordinary one anyway. It was also pointed out there that, quite apart from that problem, the principle would not even entail the conclusion that organ donation must be unpaid without the question-begging *definition* of altruism as 'unpaid'. Here the prob-lems are similar. Quite apart from the question of why altruism should be demanded at all, the way this is expressed depends on defining altruism as *impartial* selflessness, which is certainly not the usual meaning of the term—and, of course, is different from the one used in the arguments about payment.

Altruism in general is a matter of doing something for the good of another rather than oneself. If I give my sister a kidney I am in any ordinary sense of the word being altruistic (as indeed I would be if I sold it to get her something else she needed). It certainly does not require my accepting, when my sister needs a kidney, that all I can do is offer one of mine to whoever is most in need, in the hope that this pushes her nearer to the top of the list—and of course nobody expects anything of the sort. Once again, 'altruism' ap-pears as a usefully unspecific word with connotations of moral goodness that can be twisted into plausible justifications for what-ever is wanted, as long as the people hearing the arguments are not quick enough to catch the sleight of hand that is going on. My sus-picion is that the word may have first appeared in the context of donation as a way of assuring people that their organs are their own and need not be given at all, and to persuade them to agree to donate by making them feel noble about doing so. Then, as people started looking for defences of their preconceptions in other areas of the transplant debate, 'altruism', defined as whatever happened to suit the context, slipped from being a simple description of the motives of a donor into being a necessary condition of donation. The organs debate provides endless material for the analysis of politically persuasive rhetoric which amounts to intellectual cheating. Anyway, the appeal to altruism does not work in this context, any more than it did in that of organ selling—and even if it did, it could not explain why the altruism required for living donation need not be impartial, while for deceased donation it must be.

Setting aside the altruism requirement, then, the question that needs to be addressed here is simply whether all cadaveric organs should, as a matter of principle, go to the person at the top of some impartially constructed list. Is that a defensible principle?

Something like it is certainly necessary when it comes to the distribution of public goods, whose impartial allocation is essential to any decent political system. But many goods are not public, and the essence of private goods is that they are not available for impartial allocation in this way. Their disposal lies, in general, in the hands of their owners. Anyone who wants to accept a principle of impartial allocation of cadaveric organs, therefore, needs to start by arguing that they should be regarded public goods.

There is of course endless scope for dispute about how many of the goods people would like to regard as their own should be taken and treated as public. Some—extreme socialists—think all goods should come into the public category, for impartial distribution; but there seem to be rather few of them now, and most people think there should be a mixture of public and private goods. Among these, a few, as already commented, think that the organs of the deceased should automatically become public goods, to be taken over by the state for public benefit. However, this is certainly not the case at present. The debate about organ allocation, as it is now carried out, works against the background of an assumption that cadaveric organs are *not* public goods. Bodies are regarded as—effectively—the private property of the deceased and their families, and procurement for transplantation cannot go ahead against their wishes. This is the basis of all the language of altruism and gifts: the insistence that nobody has a right to deceased organs, and that people who choose to donate are noble and generous. And, as all the arguments about positive consent show, this is still widely regarded as the way things should be. Even the advocates of state requisition recognize that this is nowhere near politically feasible yet. Furthermore, recommenders of the 'fundamental principle' certainly cannot be aiming for any such situation, because part of that principle is that organs are '*given altruistically*'—and they could not be given at all unless they belonged in some sense to the givers. So part of the essence of the principle itself is that organs are to this extent *not* public property.

What this means is that anyone who wants to uphold this fundamental principle needs to argue that organs of the deceased should be treated as private goods to the extent that you can keep them to yourself—in so far as having them burnt or buried with the rest of you constitutes a way of keeping them—but that the only option for giving them away is to offer them to a public pool. And this is extremely odd. It is like saying that although you can choose whether to offer your spare time for voluntary work, you cannot choose to offer it to the local Oxfam shop. You can stay at home and twiddle your thumbs, if you like, but if you want to be useful you must make yourself available to some public agency that will send you to whomever it decides needs you most. Or, a closer analogy with posthumous organ donation, it is like saying that you may not bequeath your worldly wealth to Unicef or the Methodist Homes for the Aged. You can choose to have it buried or cremated with you, but must otherwise hand it over to the government for impartial distribution.

Not many people people, presumably, would recommend either of these curious mixtures of choice and conscription, and it is difficult to think of any other context than organ procurement where such a thing has even been proposed, let alone treated as a matter of established principle. In the absence of considerable further argument, the so-called 'fundamental principle' said to justify disallowing directed donation must be recognized as arbitrary, anomalous, at odds with all our other ideas about altruistic giving, and difficult to defend in any terms whatsoever.

Once again, it is important to stress that the question being addressed in this section is not the general one of how we should organize the collection and distribution of organs from the dead. It is quite specifically whether a particular principle—the principle of impartial distribution—should be accepted as a *constraint* on any further discussion of the use of cadaveric organs. The argument that it should not be accepted carries no direct implications for what policy there should be, any more than the claim that there is no objection of *principle* to allowing payment for organ donation carries any particular implication for what kinds of policy there should be. And just as the arguments against accepting the wrongness of organ selling as a fundamental principle do not entail that there should be an open market, so the arguments against a principle of impartial distribution as an opening constraint on discussions about cadaveric donation do not entail that everyone making a donation should be allowed to specify any conditions they please. Just as we would want to make many rules to prevent harm in legitimate organ sales, so we would want to make sure that any arrangements for directed donation were useful and manageable.

It is particularly worth noting that there are, of course, problems about directing donation that do not arise when you are thinking about leaving somebody your antique clock. Transplants can occur only under carefully controlled conditions, and the availability of suitable arrangements would necessarily limit the possibilities available to anyone who might want to express preferences about recipients. But anyone who is not bringing in as a starting principle the wrongness of allowing directed donation will try to deal with problems as they arise, rather than using them as an excuse to put a stop to any expression of personal preferences. And, as a start, even within present systems, we could easily add the donor's preferences to all the other elements in the official weighting—which, as already suggested, are a rather disparate, incommensurable, and potentially contentious collection anyway.

However, although the principle of directed donation is important, which is why it has been discussed at some length, I do not want to take the analysis of details any further here. This is because the idea might become irrelevant in the light of the next suggestion.

Impartiality of distribution 2: reciprocity

In the case of the living, it seems that just about everyone would rather have a lower statistical life expectancy than give up the absolute right not to be killed for their organs, or have them taken without consent. Most people also seem to think that we should give people the freedom not to donate their organs after death, even though this also has a cost in terms of life expectancy; and if people really would, on consideration, rather preserve their veto over the use of their dead body than increase their life expectancy by a change of rules that would make transplants more available, that also seems fair enough. The problem about the current arrangements for donation, however, is that this is not the way they work. People who are unwilling to donate do not at present lessen their own chances of receiving a transplant, because the organs available are distributed impartially among those who need them.

This suggests a different possible remedy for the ever-lengthening waiting lists. As well as trying to increase supply, we might relegate to the end of the waiting list any adult who was not willing to be on the transplantation register. And since presumably, in the long run at least, such a provision would constitute a considerable disincentive to being unavailable as a donor, such a policy could be expected to increase the donation rate considerably once established. Or, even if it did not, it would make sure that the people most likely to suffer from the unavailability of organs would be the ones not willing to give. Such an arrangement would also go along with our normal strong feelings about justice, freedom, and the need to thwart free riders. And as it would be a voluntary scheme, offering help in case of need to anyone who was willing to pay the (posthumous) cost of belonging to it, it would probably be acceptable to people who would feel quite differently about any suggestion that organs should be automatically seized by the state.

This is such an obvious idea—maximizing freedom of choice (there would still be no compulsion to be on the donor register), respecting strong feelings about ownership of bodies, and at the same time providing incentives to donate—that it is curious to consider why it has not been taken for granted from an early stage. The idea has been suggested, in one form or another, many times, and a version of it was recently adopted in Israel. My guess is that a significant part of the *explanation* is likely to be reluctance on the part of the medical profession to accept that some of their resources should come with strings attached, rather than being part of a neutral pool whose allocation they themselves control. But the *justifications* given—at least in countries committed to provision of universal health care—are usually on the lines of opposition to introducing discrimination into the health care system, and conflicting with the principle of equal rights to health care.[9] Doctors who object to any kind of directed donation or reciprocity often say it would be against their principles to allocate organs on any other basis than strict attention to need.

However, although that may be an attractive idea in itself, when it comes to the point virtually nobody will find they hold views about access to care on the basis of need in such an unqualified way. There has never been anything of the kind, except perhaps in some charitable institutions. Doctors have always been paid, usually extremely well, and in most parts of the world they are paid by individuals. They have never made a principle of treating people irrespective of payment, even though they may have done it in particular cases. And even where medical treatment is 'free at the point of delivery' it is never free to everyone: recipients have to be within the group that has collectively made such an agreement. Rights of access to benefits always have implied boundaries, and doctors are simply not in a position to say it would be against their principles to distribute anything to which they have no access to in the first place. They can allocate only what is at their disposal, and the idea that all available resources must come into this category is an illusion generated by the enlightened principles of countries that provide universal health care. In places where it is true that everyone can have access to the same resources it is because they are all part of the same taxation system—which includes the people below the tax threshold.

There are two main ways in which we organize entitlement on the basis of need. One is by specifying a group, such as the nationals or inhabitants of a country, and giving all of them access to goods such as health care on the basis of need, while at the same time requiring an appropriate contribution through taxation ('from each according to his means'). The other is to form a group of people who choose to contribute and in return have access to benefits, as in the case of private insurance. Both these methods have their defenders, but no one seems to defend the hybrid version of being able to choose not to contribute while retaining equal access to benefits, which is just the situation we have in the case of organ donation.

To this it may be objected that there are different kinds of contribution, and different kinds of need. One doctor wrote, in an online correspondence about this matter: 'we don't expect people who use bedpans to contribute bedpans; they can contribute other things'. But the trouble here is the point identified earlier: there is often no adequate substitute—or any substitute—for organs. I suppose we might consider fixing some kind of financial premium—an extra insurance contribution for people who did not want to join in the donation scheme—though that would probably be said to discriminate against people who did not want to contribute, or were too poor. But given the point that when someone needs an organ nothing else will do, my inclination is to say that people who can should provide organs. (And, for that matter, that it should be allowable to form donation insurance groups for living donation—the modified survival lottery.)

Such reciprocal arrangements, of course, remove the altruism requirement—the idea that donation is allowable only when it is a gift without expectation of return—altogether; but, as already argued, that is anomalous anyway as a fundamental principle of social organization. There are no other contexts in which desirable goods can be obtained only by altruism. What we put in its place is the willingness to make your contribution, if it turns out to be suitable when you die, in return for the corresponding willingness of other people to provide organs you may need during your life. This is just the kind of arrangement we expect all the time in other contexts, without any sense that there is anything wrong with it. In most contexts we regard this kind of arrangement as the essence of a decent society. Nobody suggests that there should be any option about paying taxes in return for social security, and any society that tried to run itself on the basis of optional taxes would soon be swept away. Total altruism is admirable, and no doubt an excellent test of fitness for heaven, but it is not a good thing to depend on for the running of a society, which is what we are concerned with here.

Of course there would be a *great deal* to be worked out in detail. We would presumably also want to make sure that people who were known in advance not to be suitable donors were included: they would be the equivalent of people too poor to pay taxes in a system of universal health care. But there would also have to be rules about such things as not allowing people to join after they had been diagnosed with a condition likely to lead to organ failure, and how to regard the status of people who had spent a long time off the register, and at what age joining the donation register should begin. However, yet again, difficulties of detail should not be mistaken for problems of principle. Here, as elsewhere, someone who accepts the principle but runs into difficulties should try to sort out the difficulties rather than abandoning the whole idea. Anyone who leaps on difficulties as an excuse to reject the whole idea is really accepting the principle of unconditionality as a constraint, and therefore needs to meet the objections given earlier.

As far as I can see, some system of reciprocity is *positively demanded* by all our normal principles about the distribution of common goods on the basis of need, and our general understanding of how a good society works: a recognition that we are all in this together, and as willing to give as to receive. If at the same time we want to allow freedom of choice about contribution, it is difficult to see what principled objection anyone could have to trying to devise a policy that restricted benefits to potential contributors—or at least gave them strong priority. It would also be very likely, in time, to increase the numbers of organs available. I think we should be trying to devise such a scheme.

Conclusion

When I began to think about these questions, I presumed, as I said earlier, that the main obstacle to procurement of enough cadaveric organs was individual conservatism and perhaps squeamishness:

deep, traditional feelings among the public about the appropriate treatment of bodies. Like most of my transplant colleagues, I thought that the only practicable way to go about getting more organs would be to do all we could to bring about a gradual shift in public opinion.

What the arguments here suggest is that if we want to increase organ donation from the dead, we need to think about matters in a much more radical way: not in terms of compulsion, at least not yet, but in terms of structural changes that would alter the framework within which individual decisions are made. And (this was the real surprise) the conservatism that resists change of *that* kind seems to lie not with the public, but more with clinicians and politicians, and probably lawyers.

Many people do have strong feelings about funerals and respect for the dead, but that seems not to be the main cause of the problem. Such feelings are probably the immediate cause of family refusal, but the reason for families being involved in donation decisions at all is that we have not yet adapted the system of organ donation to our general principles of managing death, which separate the disposal of bodies and the disposal of property. If we recognized donation as being an aspect of bequests, not of the care of the dead that has always been the responsibility of the family, that would clarify the matter. Family consent would not be needed where the deceased had made the appropriate arrangements for donation. If that were settled as a matter of law, we could begin to think more clearly about how to organize the practice.

That in itself, of course, would not make anyone more willing to donate organs. But it would be much easier to address the problem of how to increase donation if we started from the way we normally think about other property. We could then consider arrangements such as a system of reciprocity, and possibly some directing of donation, either of which would be likely to change the way people thought about the matter. It is also most unlikely that the public would oppose any such changes, because they are so much in line with the way people think of their rights over their own bodies anyway.

Here is how we might approach the matter in the light of what has been argued so far.

First, then, the development of transplantation means that the status of deceased organs has changed radically. Their transferability makes them valuable commodities, and that means we need rules to govern their transference from one person to another.

Furthermore, the way organs are spoken about shows that they are naturally regarded as *belonging* to the person whose organs they are. This is shown in all kinds of ways. In official quarters it appears in the pervasive language of gifts and altruism to encourage donation. It also seems to show in the way people had no objection to the incineration of discarded tissues and organs, but objected very strongly whenever they discovered that these had been taken, without consent, for use by other people. This suggests that the most natural way to think about them is as property, and in the first instance belonging to the person whose organs they are.

At the moment bodies and body parts are not legally property, and it is easy to see why this was traditionally so. But that was when body parts were generally of no use except as parts of functioning wholes. Given that people already intuitively seem to regard their body parts as theirs, and that something very close to this idea is already entrenched in laws and practices about consent to donation, there is no reason for not recognizing the matter formally. We should overcome the 'commodification' emotion—which takes its negative connotations from quite different contexts—and clarify things by making organs legally the property of the person whose organs they are, or, in this case, were. My guess is that this would be regarded as entirely appropriate by the public—especially as it would, at least prima facie, reinforce the feeling that nobody had the right to take your organs without consent. It is hard to imagine anyone complaining about their organs being formally declared *their property*.

However, although such a change would not actually entail any particular policies about the procurement of organs, it would involve some shift of perception. In particular, it would suggest a presumption in favour of working on the basis of normal inferences from property rights, and people's being able to do with organs the kinds of thing they could do with other things they owned. This presumption would probably need modifying in various ways, since organs for transplant have characteristics that mean they need special treatment, but it would be the appropriate starting position. In the case of the dead, therefore, the natural starting point would be the way we deal with other property of deceased persons. We should start by following established principles that determine whether anyone else inherits them, and if so who. The bequest of organs could not depend on the legal processes involved in wills in the way that other property does, because of the speed and technological skill needed for transplantation; there would need to be readily available databases for finding out what provisions people had made. But the arrangements would have to be legally binding in the way wills are, and not overridable by relatives.

Again, it seems likely that most people would agree that the properly formulated instructions of individuals should be paramount in cases of conflict with the wishes of relatives. There would be no loss to people with strong family ties: they could leave their organs to the family for decisions about donation, or make the decisions in agreement with them before death. That would settle the principle of family involvement (with plenty of scope for people who disagreed with their families), and allow for the formal separation of donation and disposal. Relatives should not even be consulted about donation. This all looks intuitively feasible too, at least from a legal point of view.

Of course the practicalities would still present problems, since it is much more difficult to pass on organs in a useful way than it is to pass on ordinary objects. But if the principle were accepted, the experts who understand both dying and organ retrieval could put their minds to devising the best ways to achieve the smooth management of both. In principle it should make things easier for clinical teams, because there would be no discussion of organ retrieval with the family. If that aspect of matters were handled by a separate team, the clinicians who had been caring for the patient could give all their attention to the family. The family's concern could be restored to death and disposal, as it always had been.

It would be good to make sure that as many people as possible declared their wishes in the appropriate way, but, just as in the case of other possessions, it would be necessary to make provisions for intestacy. Many of us (the natural opters-out and requisitionists) would prefer it if suitable organs for which no provision had been made were used automatically for transplant, as in hard opting-out arrangements. But this would obviously be a matter to be decided by the public, and it probably would not be acceptable yet. If so, the natural default, as in other areas of intestacy, would be for the decision to pass to the family. In some ways this would not be very different from current opting-in procedures, since where the decedent had not made specific provisions the family would decide in any case. But it would be slightly better from the point of view of procurement, since following the usual pattern of inheritance would make it clear which member of the family was the heir. I gather that at present, when the family makes collective decisions about donation, any negative voice tends to prevail.

Regarding organs as being in the same legal category as other bequests would, however, suggest considerable changes in other respects. There would be no objection whatever *in principle* to directed donation. Organs could be specified as going to family members or friends if they needed them, or to particular groups with whom the decedent felt particular sympathy, or, of course, bequeathed as now for general availability. There would also be no prima facie objection to other possibilities at present looked at askance by many people, such as accepting money for funeral expenses in return for donation of organs. As this would facilitate much better funerals and memorials for many people, it might well be seen—once donation and disposal were recognized as distinct—as a positive way of honouring the dead. And there would also be no objection to systems of reciprocity, which also would probably encounter no public resistance whatever because they are so much in line with all our normal feelings about fairness and the conduct of good societies.

However, this is still all at the level of principle. It is most important to stress this: the arguments presented here have been about the idea that unconditionality of donation should not be treated as a *constraint* on the discussion of policy. Even if there is no objection of principle to directed donation, there would inevitably be strong constraints of practicality. Once again, bequeathing organs cannot be like bequeathing most other possessions, because they have to be collected, preserved, and transferred. What anyone could use-fully achieve by bequeathing organs would depend on the arrange-ments available. And here is a whole new subject, because the availability of medical expertise is so variable, and a massive moral and political question in its own right. Personally, I am all for doing as much as possible through public policy rather than free enter-prise, but obviously issues of that scale cannot possibly be analysed as a subsection of a book on transplantation. All I can do here is mark an area for investigation of a quite different kind, whose reso-lution in different countries might result in quite different possi-bilities for organ donation and transfer, depending on whether the overall framework was one of free enterprise or a centrally organ-ized system that offered health care to everyone, or any combina-tion of the two.

For countries or states with universal provision, the best ar-rangement would probably be a system of reciprocity, with a common pool to which individuals would be asked to contribute their organs, for impartial distribution, when they died. This need not necessarily be the only possible way of making a useful be-quest; everything would depend on the background arrangements. Again, it is difficult to imagine any public objection to the setting up of such a system, since it leaves everyone free to make their own decision, and is so strongly in line with ordinary feelings about fair-ness. Even if we have strong feelings about who should benefit from what we have to give, we also seem to have a deep under-standing of reciprocal altruism, and the appropriateness of being willing to make contributions to other people's well-being if they are willing to contribute to ours. And if there were such a pool, and if willingness to bequeath organs to that pool would significantly increase an individual's chance of getting organs if they were needed, it might not be long before most people chose to join in. A few headlines about people who had died because their unwilling-ness to donate had left them a long way down the waiting list might well make a considerable difference to public attitudes.

This matter would, of course, connect with the opting in and out problem—now translated into problems about will-making and intestacy. Many people do not get around to making a will, and it would be very serious if people who had kept intending to join the scheme, but not quite doing it, unexpectedly found themselves in need of a transplant and too far down the list to have much chance of getting one. This suggests that in a system of reciprocity the de-fault should be that everyone was part of it. This would be a matter for public debate, but it might well make a considerable difference to attitudes. It would be ideal to make sure through the general medical system that everyone had specified a preference one way or the other, but most people would probably agree that, for anyone who did slip through the net, it would be better for their organs to be used without explicit consent after their death than for them to discover when they turned out to need a transplant that they were significantly less likely to get one than people who had registered.

However, the question of what arrangements would turn out to be best is not the issue here. My general claim is that although nothing like enough people are choosing to donate under present circumstances, and that although public opinion seems to demand that people should have choice about the use of their deceased organs, that is not the end of the matter. What we should be looking at is the institutional arrangements that have the effect of *limiting* people's choices, and which are *not* in place because of the insistence of the public. These obstructions are rooted in legal and medical tradition, and apparently kept in place because of the conservatism of their practitioners, and of politicians who regard those practitioners as the relevant experts. Even though not enough people are choosing to donate in the present system, it does not follow that they would refuse to accept radical changes in the system, which would themselves almost certainly result in more procurement of organs from the dead. If these arguments have been right, the deepest problems lie not in people's possessiveness about their own bodies, but in legal and medical traditions *that have no justification* in terms of our normal values and the present state of technology. There is no justification for not regarding organs as the property of the people whose organs they are, and following through the implications of that recognition. Such a change might make an enormous, relatively uncontroversial, difference to the rate of organ procurement.

And although this chapter is specifically about procurement from the dead, it is worth commenting that recognition of organs as property would also change the emphasis of discussions about transfer of organs from the living. The argument of this chapter has been that many of the problems of deceased donation arise because the background arrangements—in which the family is naturally in charge of disposal of the dead—fit uneasily with the new reality of organs as transferable goods. The same is true in the case of the living. We are still dealing with living donation essentially as a case of giving consent for treatment, which, as already established, is difficult to square with the idea that medical treatment is supposed to be for the benefit of the patient, while in this case the treatment involved does direct harm. Once again, however, it is clear that people do think of their organs as their property, as is shown by the spontaneous development of organ selling, and it also appears in the familiar official language of gifts. There is no good reason for not accepting them formally and legally as property. It would not directly imply that organs should be regarded in all respects like all other property. There are already many ways in which particular categories of property (such as antiquities and works of art) are subject to special provisions, and in the same way special regulations could apply to the transfer of organs from the living—such as, perhaps, limiting the amount of harm that could be inflicted even with consent. But a change to recognizing organs as property would also emphasize that the default should be regarding them as transferable property owned by the person in whose body they were, and that justification needed to be given for any reason for additional restrictions. Again, it seems unlikely that many people would object to their being told that their organs were legally their property, and under their control.[†]

[†] It would also be interesting to see what happened if the question of an absolute prohibition of payment were expressed not in terms of the rich as predators of the poor, but of individuals' own entitlement to accept payment for a living donation, and what safeguards they thought should be in place to protect anyone who made such a choice. Although most people certainly do react with horror to the idea of organ selling when they hear of it, it is significant that the immediate, total ban was not a response to public pressure, but again

In sum, therefore, the matter seems to me to be more or less this. Transplantation has developed in a framework of arrangements that were not designed for it. Within this framework, not enough people choose to donate, and everyone seems reluctant to resort to compulsion. But we have been working on the basis of nothing more than piecemeal adjustments to the background systems, and we need to think at a more radical level. Different arrangements in law and institutional organization could considerably alter the way we approached detailed questions of policies and arrangements, and as a result the availability of organs. Furthermore, these more radical changes would probably not be opposed, but welcomed, by the public.[10]

If so, the deepest problems about procurement of organs from the dead lies not in the conservatism of the public, as is generally presumed, but in that of the medical and legal professions and the politicians. That is an interesting, startling thought.

came from politicians and the profession. It would be interesting to find out more about public attitudes to the issue in a study that took care to separate the objection of principle from questions about policies and safeguards.

5

PENUMBRAL PROBLEMS

Life before death

Even if we had all the issues of consent for organ donation sorted out, there would still remain one enormous problem about the procurement of organs after death. People who are entirely happy about donation, and have not the slightest objection to the posthumous use of their organs, may nevertheless be concerned about what being recognized as a prospective donor might imply for life before death.

Transplant centres cannot work just by collecting bodies after people have died. Although the donors must be dead, the organs to be transplanted need to be as alive as possible—as already noted, living kidney donations do better than cadaveric ones—and organ deterioration after death, left to itself, is very rapid. If organs of the dead are to be used at all, work to preserve and use them must begin at the earliest possible moment. This means that, with hardly any exceptions, suitable donors are people who die in hospital under circumstances where the transplant team can get straight into action. Collecting and maintaining parts from the dead and transferring them to the living are all part of a continuous process demanding high skill and specialist equipment, and the process must be unbroken.

This does at least mean that there is no scope for present-day versions of the enterprising amateurs who supplied nineteenth-century anatomists with their corpses. We are not going to be murdered or dug out of our graves by opportunists with ideas of turning up at the doors of transplant units and offering bodies for sale. But still, there is plenty of scope for other kinds of anxiety. In countries with advanced medical systems many of us will in fact be in hospital when we eventually die, because hospitals are where seriously ill people are now taken as a matter of routine. If the people supposed to be responsible for keeping us alive are closely and essentially linked with the ones who are trying to collect spare parts for keeping other people alive, it is hardly surprising if the transplant programme is regarded with suspicion by many people.

It is in the management of dying patients that the colliding interests of donors and recipients are at their sharpest. When we go into hospital, most people—probably all—want to be absolutely sure that their treatment will be entirely directed to their own interests, and not the interests of their organs' posthumous value to other people. But how can we be sure about this? The people treating us know what they are doing, but we and our non-expert families and friends probably do not. Might the clinicians supposedly looking after us be surreptitiously bent on achieving other ends? People who know about the recent history of medicine may know that—within the memory of some currently practising doctors—patients were routinely used as research subjects, and even subjected to treatments that had nothing to do with their own condition, because the doctors involved could pass off their experiments as part of the treatment. If incoming hospital patients can be identified as potential donors, might they not receive treatment directed more towards the interests of their transplantable organs than of themselves, without their even being aware of it?

From the point of view of technical possibilities, unconstrained by law and ethics, there are many things clinicians could do to increase your value as a prospective organ donor once they had you in their hands. They could, at the very least, give you medication or treatment that did not actually harm you, but whose purpose was to preserve your organs for the purposes of transplantation. They could decide against your continued treatment, declaring it futile or not in your interests, in the hope that you would die so that your organs became available. Perhaps they might even deliberately kill you, or (much the same in practice) cut corners by declaring you dead before it was absolutely certain that you were, and start taking your organs while you were still alive. Being in the hands of experts whose trades you do not understand, and whose interests may not be identical with your own, is bad enough when you are dealing with plumbers and car mechanics. The prospect of being in the hands of experts in the human machine, and furthermore trapped on their premises, may well seem to many of us seriously alarming.

There certainly are some people—presumably no one knows how many—whose fears of this kind make them reluctant to be on any donor list. They have no objection to being deceased donors, but they want to be sure that deceased is what they actually will be, and only after all worthwhile efforts have been made to keep them alive. Some people do say that if an opting-out system were established they would indeed opt out, not because they would object to being donors, but because they are afraid of what might happen if they could be recognized before death as potential donors. (The most recent person from whom I heard this was himself a transplant professional.) They would be quite happy for their relatives to give consent after their death, but not to be identifiable as donors in advance.

This is something of which people in the transplant community are acutely aware, and whenever they discuss the question of how to increase donation rates there is endless talk of the importance of establishing trust, and great anxiety about anything that might be presented by scandalmongering journalists and bloggers as cause for alarm. Many of them still talk in horror about a 1980 BBC *Panorama* programme that stirred up doubts as to whether deceased donors were really dead. Public trust is essential to the whole enterprise, and an absolute requirement of most people is that they should be safe in the hands of the medical profession. This is probably another of the things most people regard as mattering far more than any increase in statistical life expectancy that might result from clinicians' stretching a point here and there towards the end of life in the interests of procurement. If so, the success of the transplant project—at least in a democracy—will depend on people's being given adequate assurance that their interests will be given absolute priority.

This is a complicated matter, because problems of trust come at several different levels. At the top—the surface layer—there is the need to persuade people that they are in safe hands. This is a matter of public relations, and obviously of great importance. Being trustworthy and appearing so are not the same, and if the aim is reassurance, simply being trustworthy is not enough on its own.

Second, there is the matter of making sure that the people involved in transplantation, at all levels, actually are trustworthy. This largely depends on the culture of the profession, and the extent to which practitioners and their ruling bodies exert vigilance for aberrant individuals and slipping standards. Obviously groups of people can get together and conspire against outsiders, and although doctors sometimes talk as though there has been an unbroken tradition of high standards of medical ethics—selfless consideration of people in need and total integrity—not much knowledge of the history of medicine is needed to show that standards of ethics have varied enormously over time and between places. Nor is much understanding of human nature needed to suggest that doctors are likely to be as variable in their personal and cultural moral standards as any other group.*

* In particular, hospitals have traditions of their own, and for most of history they were only the last resort of people who could not afford to pay for medical treatment at home. Until relatively recently nothing more could be done for you in hospital than at home by a visiting doctor, and hospital doctors certainly did not regard patients in anything like the way they are supposed to regard them now. Patients had to be thankful for anything they could get, while doctors could do pretty well what they liked with them; and the culture persisted, albeit in increasingly attenuated form, for a long time. Until quite recently—well within living memory—many doctors expected their patients to be passive recipients of care, to be treated without consultation or explanation, and in that kind of atmosphere all sorts of things could go on without patients' knowing. The medical experiments on unconsulted patients, mentioned earlier, were already in direct contravention of the widely accepted policies expressed in the Nuremberg Declaration (1947) and the Declaration of Helsinki (1961) about research on human subjects, but groups of doctors had cultures of their own and carried on for a long time with no external constraints. So if patients in hospital have doubts about whether they can rely on being treated in their own interests, they have a good deal of history on their side.

However, those aspects of trust are essentially practical, organizational matters. Here my concern is with a deeper level of problem. We might have total trust in medical organizations and individual clinicians to follow all the established rules of law and professional ethics, but unless those rules themselves provided the necessary protection, there would still be inadequate grounds for confidence. What we need to sort out first, at the foundation of this complex edifice of trust, is what kinds of rule—in law and professional ethical standards—would actually provide patients with adequate protection against premature use as organ donors. That is the first question for any systematic enquirer into the subject.

There are some people who argue that the standards currently accepted in law and medical practice involve restrictions that go far beyond anything needed for the protection of patients, and that we should be relaxing them in the interests of increased organ procurement. But there are also others who argue that we have already gone too far, and that current standards allow doctors to take organs before they should. These are the questions to be addressed here.

Current constraints

Transplant surgery came into a world in which there was already a mass of law to protect the living; and living is, of course, what potential donors are even while they are dying. Until people are actually dead, they are regarded as having all the fundamental rights of the living. They have all the negative rights that protect them from being killed or harmed, and as long as they are competent they may not even be inappropriately touched or otherwise intruded on without their consent. Patients in hospitals also have many positive rights, because the institutions and the people who work in them have duties of care towards them.

This means that none of the things people are afraid of, when they think about being used prematurely as sources of organs, are actually allowed in law or by professional standards. You certainly cannot be killed. Treatment can be withdrawn if it is regarded as futile or not in your interests, but it can never be withdrawn *so that* you will die and be available as a donor. As long you are competent no treatment at all may be given without your fully informed consent, and that rules out surreptitious medication on behalf of any future recipients of your organs. If you are not competent, any treatment given must be in your own interests. Your death cannot be actively hastened,[†] or your organs taken before you are dead.

Although the existence of rules, as already remarked, is in itself no guarantee that they will be followed, it is also worth pointing out that at least in parts of the world with strong institutional controls over medical provision there are many pressures to make sure these guarantees really are met. In the case of transplants, furthermore, there are extra safeguards. The clinicians responsible for the care of patients are entirely separate from the transplant team, and the transplanters have no say in judgements about the treatment of patients who might become donors. Patients can also take comfort from the fact that doctors do not like their patients to die, since that in itself is a kind of failure, and also in the inevitable tension resulting from the fact that there is a sense in which the transplanters'

[†] You may be treated in ways that have the incidental effect of shortening your life if there is a genuinely therapeutic purpose, such as pain relief.

success is dependent on the life-saving failure of their colleagues in the intensive care units. As commented earlier, this does not mean the two groups are always at odds in practice—ideally, and often in reality, there is careful cooperation—but the potential for conflict and rivalry provides an extra safeguard for patients who may be anxious about premature treatment as organ farms. Patients themselves are also increasingly well informed, and they and their relatives can consult the Internet to find out what is going on and monitor it. And the eagerness of journalists to sniff out scandals (genuine or spurious) and enterprising lawyers to look out promising cases for compensation claims, as well as the anxiety of transplanters themselves to keep public opinion on their side and not to do anything that will have the tabloid press pricking up its ears, provides yet another layer of safeguards. So if all this is true, we may think everything is just as it should be. People who are adequately informed should realize there is nothing to worry about.

There is, however, such a thing as leaning over backwards. Although everyone seems to agree that we should give total protection to potential organ donors, the anxiety about adverse reactions already makes it overwhelmingly more likely that transplant organs will be lost unnecessarily than taken inappropriately. Overcautious concern about dying patients and their families, and what will happen if there is any hint of scandal, already leads to the unnecessary loss of organs whose retrieval and use would be perfectly allowable within the present legal framework. But also, more than this, it is being argued by some people that the rules themselves are stronger than is actually needed, and protect what needs no protection.

The starting presumption in favour of getting transplant organs whenever possible can again be used to test the restrictions that currently obstruct procurement. The question about any such restriction will be whether the protection it is supposed to provide for the living is really of any value to them.

Treatment in the patient's interests

The first rule that is open to this sort of challenge is that all treatment must be in the patient's interests. This means not just that treatment must not be *against* the patient's interests; it must be positively in them. Even if you would do no harm to living patients by treating them in the interests of a potential organ recipient, you must not do this without their consent.

At least on the face of it, this sounds entirely appropriate. If we had been in hospital and found out afterwards that some of our treatment had really been for the benefit of someone else, without our consent, most of us would probably be appalled even if assured that it had done no harm to us. However, no one is suggesting any modification of the rules that demand informed consent from competent patients. The real issues arise in the case of non-competent patients.

Consider, for instance, such circumstances as these:

1. A young man is unconscious and dying on a general ward. Nothing more can be done for him, and there is no possibility of his ever recovering consciousness. On the other hand, by the time he dies, if he remains where he is, his organs will have deteriorated to the point of uselessness for transplantation. If he were moved to

intensive care, and kept on a ventilator until his death, the organs could be kept in a viable state.

This procedure—'elective ventilation'—was proposed, and formulated in the UK as 'The Exeter Protocol' by clinicians who thought it was reasonable to act in this way because it could do the relevant patients absolutely no harm, in terms either of comfort or of life expectancy, and would potentially save the lives of many others. But when the Department of Health sought legal opinion about the matter, the advice was that it was probably unlawful because the treatment was not directed to the interests of the patients themselves. On that basis, the Department of Health ruled against it.

2. A patient on a ventilator is dying and terminally unconscious, but not yet brain-dead. There is no chance of recovery, and therefore continuing ventilation is not in the patient's interests. Ventilation counts as treatment, and therefore according to the law it should be discontinued and the patient left to die unventilated. But, once again, death away from the ventilator will mean that the organs are less useful, or even useless, for transplant purposes. If the patient could go on being ventilated until death the organs would be usable.

In neither of these cases would the ventilation do any harm to the dying patient—who would never be aware of it, or of anything else—and in both situations it would mean that many other lives could be saved. To many people it seems that we should obviously allow ventilation in these circumstances, and that the rules preventing it go far beyond what is needed for the protection of the patient. It is true that in cases of the second kind the matter can in fact often be fudged in practice, because there is no clear criterion for when ventilation has definitely ceased to be in a patient's interests: families often want treatment to carry on because they are 'hoping for a miracle', and doctors are anxious to show that they are doing everything possible. Nevertheless, if they believe the treatment has no hope of doing the patient any good, it is technically illegal to continue with it. And anyway, people who are anxious to increase the pool of transplant organs do not want to have to rely on fudges.

Some people who are worried by the waste of organs in contexts like these have tried to get round the problem by arguing that the necessary procedures might be allowable even under current law, at least in cases where the dying patient has already expressed willingness to be an organ donor. One such suggestion is that since competent patients can give advance refusal for treatment in case they later become incompetent, they should also be regarded as able to give advance consent, and that consent for organ donation amounts to tacit consent for whatever procedures are necessary to achieve this end. But although the idea of tacit consent is in itself legitimate, I gather lawyers do not think much of this argument, and most people would probably agree with them. If you consent to my staying in your house while you are away, and I forget to bring the key, it does not seem to follow that you have tacitly consented to my breaking down the door. Something on these lines could obviously be arranged, however, so it is at least worth considering when we are designing the arrangements under which people consent to donation.

Another such line of argument is that if you take a wide enough interpretation of what constitutes someone's interests, you can count preservation of organs for donation as actually being in the interests of the donor. This is perhaps more promising, as it does seem to be in line with trends in recent incapacity law, which interprets a person's interests as encompassing what the person's wishes were before competence was lost. So perhaps there is some chance there; it would be interesting to test it. It certainly sounds like something we should be arguing for. Whether or not more radical reforms can be justified and implemented, we should in the meantime go on doing everything we can to increase donation by means of nudges at the edges of the present law.

Nevertheless, even if either of these stratagems could be made to work in law, their scope would still be limited to people who had registered as donors, or whose positive wishes to donate were known by other means. The argument that it should be regarded as in such people's interests to be treated in ways that enhanced their usefulness as organ donors—at least as long as it did not harm them in other ways—is certainly one we should be pressing; but it could not be used in the case of patients whose wishes were not known (but whose relatives might be willing to consent), or even ones who might be involved in some possible reciprocity arrangement. Those cases would still not allow for organ-preserving treatment against the background of a rule that treatment must always be positively in the patient's interests. Surely, it might be argued, it is wrong to allow organs in such cases to be lost, at great cost, without any corresponding benefit to anyone?

There are two kinds of proposal that might be made here to avoid this loss without giving prospective donors anything to worry about. One is that it should be regarded as acceptable to treat non-competent people in ways that were not positively in their interests as long as the treatment was not *against* their interests. This version is likely to arouse a lot of concern because most people seem to feel that as patients they want nothing but their own interests to be taken into account when treatment decisions are made—though that does not mean the idea is not worth considering. However, a less extreme position would be to argue that rules about acting in the patient's interests become irrelevant when the patient no longer *has* any relevant interests—and that this can often occur before the patient is actually dead. When patients are terminally unconscious, as in the cases described above—when they cannot possibly be brought back to consciousness before they die—their own interests as living beings have already ended, and there is therefore no more possibility of acting in those interests than against them. They may still have interests in any sense in which the dead have interests, such as having their wishes carried out, but not the interests of living people.

If some such principle were adopted it would allow for organ retrieval in the cases outlined above, because a *terminally unconscious* patient has no interests that could be harmed by elective ventilation,[1] and, furthermore, no interests that could be advanced by any other treatment. Of course many people would object strongly to any such suggestion, because they regard as fundamental the principle that the full rights of the living must be respected for the whole of life, and that no modification of this principle should ever be allowed. I shall discuss that later. For now the intention is just clarification, and identifying the issue as one that needs to be addressed by anyone thinking through these problems.

The prohibition of killing and the dead donor rule

The second problem raised by people who are concerned about the waste of viable organs lies in a principle that sounds even further beyond question than the principle of treating only in the interests of the patient: the prohibitions on killing and on taking organs before a prospective donor is actually dead. The proposals for change here again concern patients who are terminally unconscious, but, in these cases, ones whose organs cannot be maintained by ventilation during the dying process. By the time they do die, their organs will have deteriorated beyond use. At present, however, it is not allowable either to speed up death deliberately, because that would be murder, or to start taking organs before the person is dead ('the dead donor rule').

Here are two such cases:

3. A young man is in a permanent vegetative state. He has been in this state for two years, but he is breathing normally and is being maintained by artificial nutrition and hydration (ANH). He could continue in this state for many years, but scans show no activity at all in his upper brain. He is completely unconscious, and as the upper brain has become liquid throughout, with no remaining structure, there is no chance of his ever recovering consciousness. An application is made to the courts to discontinue ANH and allow him to die, and this is granted. But the resulting death by slow dehydration will leave his organs beyond use. If the organs could be taken as soon as the decision to discontinue treatment had been made, or death brought forward, the organs could be used. Since the patient is terminally unconscious this would make no difference whatever to him, but it would make a huge difference to all the people whose lives could be saved.

4. A woman with severe head damage is on a ventilator and terminally unconscious but not yet brain-dead, and she could live for some time if ventilation continued. Ventilation is no longer in her

interests, so it should by law be stopped. Even if that constraint could be got round, however, death might still be some time away. The intensive care resources cannot be spared indefinitely, and even if they could there would almost certainly be organ damage or deterioration by the time death occurred. When the decision is made to end ventilation, the patient will be returned to the wards and will probably die very soon afterwards. In an increasing number of hospitals arrangements are in place to collect any organs that can still be used under such circumstances (NHBD—non-heart-beating donation). But the organs will still deteriorate during the dying process, and many if not all will become unusable, or at least less valuable. It would be better from the point of view of organ donation to take the organs while the patient was still on the ventilator. Since the patient is terminally unconscious, she will never know anything about it either way.

The proposal that we should abandon the so-called 'dead donor rule' in such cases has been made, but not widely pressed.[2] People who have reached the conclusion that doing so would be morally justified—indeed morally required—also think there is very little chance of overcoming the general idea that killing people to get their organs, or plundering their bodies for organs before they are dead—which amounts to much the same thing[3]—is straightfor-wardly murder. Still, this is a question that needs to be addressed by anyone thinking through the ethics of organ procurement. Of course taking organs while people are actually alive, even though permanently unconscious, goes against immediate intuitive reac-tions as well as current law and professional standards. There are deep feelings of resistance to direct killing in normal circumstances, and in countries where euthanasia is allowed many doctors who practise it nevertheless admit to feeling a strong reluctance to kill, and have to keep in mind their conviction of its moral necessity to be able to do it. But, once again, the question is about justification. Should the absolute prohibition on killing be kept in place even when it makes no difference to the person killed, and could result in the saving of several other lives?

No doubt many people will come to the conclusion that there should be no change in our present standards, and that as long as life persists, so should all the currently accepted rights of the living.

Still, even if it is accepted that either direct killing or hastening death through organ removal should be out of the question, whether for reasons of deep morality or of public relations, the same problem is nevertheless forcing itself on us from a different direction. Transplantation has confronted us with a particularly acute version of the ancient problem of how we can really be sure that someone is dead.

Recognizing death

Most people around us are obviously, beyond question, alive. Others, not seen by any of us most of the time, are equally obviously dead. Sometimes it is quite clear when someone has just made the transition between the two states. Nevertheless, there have always been cases in which there is some reasonable doubt about whether a person is alive or dead. All the obvious signs of life, such as breathing, movement, and response to stimuli seem to have gone, but occasionally people in that kind of state have been known to return. That means—unless there is a known miracle worker on hand—that they were not really dead in spite of the fact that they seemed to be. So how can we be sure when someone really is dead?

The way societies have coped with the problem has always been to err on the side of caution. There is a massive difference in moral and legal status between the living and the dead, and nobody doubts that it is better to risk treating people as alive when they are dead than treating them as dead when they are alive. It is much better to leave the dead unburied until you are absolutely certain than to risk burying the living.

At what stage of deterioration this certainty could be reached has depended on the state of knowledge. Traditionally you might suspect death when, perhaps, there was not enough breath to disturb a feather or mist a mirror, but still not think you could reasonably treat the person as dead until the body started going cold and stiff—or even started to putrefy. You waited, in effect, until the body had got into a state from which nobody had ever been known to return, and then you could be sure the person was dead.

Waiting for a few hours or even days in this way did not matter much as long as all you needed to do was to pass on property, or proclaim the next king, or plan a funeral. Nothing serious or irreversible needed to be done immediately to the person who seemed to be dead. But transplantation has changed this, and brought a new urgency to the problem of establishing death. Any time you spend waiting to be sure that the person is dead is time when deterioration will progress; and the further it progresses, the less chance there is of the organs being of much, if any, use when you eventually do decide that death is beyond doubt. For the purposes of transplantation you need to start preserving organs as early as possible; and if you are not allowed to start any organ retrieval or preservation before death, you need to be able to recognize death the moment it happens.

Of course science has progressed a long way since the days when it was necessary to wait for bodies to be cold and stiff. Once the circulation of the blood had been discovered, and the function of heart and lungs understood, it was clear that there was no possibility of any recovery after the cardio-pulmonary system had closed down. You could safely take cessation of heartbeat as the point of no return, and that meant that you could confidently declare death at a much earlier point in the closing-down process than had been possible before. Any other goings-on in the body, such as warmth, twitching, and continuing evidence of digestion, which before would have been regarded as evidence that life still lingered and might possibly return, could be seen as residual after-effects of life rather than as an indication that life remained. Death could be declared with confidence at a much earlier stage. And, of course, science has gone enormously further since that was established. There is now far more understanding of which parts of the system depend on which others, and there are monitors to detect the slightest flicker of anything. So surely, we might think, pinpointing the exact moment of death should now be easier than ever. But, paradoxically, these huge scientific and technological advances have actually made the whole problem more difficult.

One aspect of the difficulty is raised by the sensitivity of the various monitors. When you have only crude methods of observation you cannot see much about the details of how the different parts of the system are closing down in relation to each other. As far as you can see without specialist equipment, breathing and heartbeat come to an end pretty well simultaneously, and you can regard them as a single unit. Now, however, it is possible to observe the different elements separately, and see the exact order of their closing down in particular cases. This would not be of much practical significance on its own, however: the elements are still closely enough connected to make no difference from the point of view of transplants, because by the time any question of procurement arises both will have ceased, and the order of their ending does not matter. The real trouble comes in the fact that we can not only recognize the details of how the system is working and see what is going on, but also intervene in it.

This is, of course, just what medicine is supposed to do. When parts of the system are naturally interlinked, so that when one fails others rapidly follow, we can often stimulate processes or damp them down, mend broken parts, remove malignant ones, and even replace totally failing ones with mechanical devices or transplants. If you have total kidney failure you will, left to the workings of nature, be dead after a painful struggle in a few days. If, on the other hand, you are put on a dialysis machine, or given a transplant, kidney failure and death can be drawn far apart. With appropriate treatment, you can now survive the death of your kidneys by years or decades—and of course there is no doubt that you are alive even though your original kidneys are not. But the same kind of separation can now be achieved between the elements whose more or less simultaneous failure had been recognized as constituting death, and that is where the trouble comes.

The serious problem for the identification of death came with the development of the mechanical ventilator. Artificial ventilation was first developed in the 1950s during a major polio epidemic, when patients were dying because their lungs were paralysed. It was realized that if breathing could be maintained artificially until the illness passed, complete recovery was possible. This principle is still the basic idea of the intensive care unit: failing parts of the system are taken over artificially, in the hope that if the body can be helped through the crisis it will eventually recover enough to carry on alone. For the first time, it was possible to have total failure of the lungs that was not immediately followed, as a result of anoxia, by failure of the heart and the brain.

This was a great advance for medicine, but like nearly all advances it raised new difficulties of its own. One obvious problem was that decisions had to be made about how long to persist with ventilation if recovery was unlikely, or if such recovery as might be possible seemed not worth achieving. But a quite different kind of problem came with a category of patients identified as being in a state of *coma dépassé*—'beyond coma'—which is now known as brain-death. It was not just *unlikely* that these patients would be able to breathe without the ventilator; it was absolutely certain that they would not, because the necessary connections between the brain and the rest of the body—in the brain stem—had completely stopped working, and there was no possibility of recovery. These patients had no chance whatever of recovering either spontaneous breathing or consciousness, but by the cardio-pulmonary criterion they were not yet dead, because the heart and lungs were still working. Without the ventilator they would have been obviously dead long before, but while ventilation continued their bodies were still functioning in many ways as normal. They still looked alive—warm and pink—with digestion and excretion still going on as normal, and in one case a foetus was even brought to term in a woman in this state. What, then, was the status of these patients? Were they being kept alive by the ventilator ('life support machine'), or was the machine pumping oxygenated blood round a corpse?

This was an important question for several reasons. In some parts of the world, for instance, discontinuing life-sustaining treatment was regarded as killing, so unless the patient was already dead, switching off the ventilator would count as wrongful killing. In other places it was legally permissible to discontinue treatment regarded as 'futile' and of no benefit to the patient, and in these places there was no problem about turning the ventilator off and allowing the patient to die. The possibility of transplantation, however, raised a quite new problem. As long as these patients remained on the ventilator many of their organs could be kept in good condition, and could be taken and used for transplantation while the ventilator was still operating. But if they were alive this was not permissible: you cannot remove the organs of a living person (the dead donor rule). On the other hand if you took the patients off the ventilator and waited for cardiac arrest, the organs would deteriorate during the process of dying and become of far less use, or useless.

This was a serious problem, and in 1967 what became known as the Ad Hoc Committee of the Harvard Medical School recommended a radical solution. If a patient's brain had died—closed down beyond any possibility of recovery that would allow return of consciousness or spontaneous breathing— the *person* had gone, and that should constitute sufficient grounds for a declaration of death, even though cardio-pulmonary function was being maintained by the ventilator. There should now be another criterion for recognizing death, in addition to the cardio-pulmonary standard. Either should be regarded as sufficient.

This recommendation has now been widely accepted, and organs from heart-beating donors—ones whose brains have died but whose circulation is being maintained by ventilation—are the basis of most cadaveric transplantation. But it has not been universally accepted. In some jurisdictions brain-dead patients on ventilators are regarded as still alive; and even in places where they are legally counted as dead many people doubt that they are *really* dead, and wonder whether the new criterion is just a fudge by transplanters to get round the dead donor rule. Even people who have no qualms in theory may find themselves uncomfortable in practice. There is a great deal of uncertainty in the minds not only of the public but also of many clinical professionals. It is common to hear of people's being declared brain-dead, and then having the ventilator switched off 'to allow them to die in peace'. 'Twice dead', as Margaret Lock says;[4] and in most people's conception death is not a kind of thing that can occur twice. If you are dead, that is the end of the matter; if there is death to follow, you were not dead in the first place.

Here lies the second set of problems mentioned earlier in the chapter, about current laws and practices of organ retrieval. While some people think that the protection offered to living donors has overreached itself, and is now preventing procurement in ways that go far beyond any kind of protection needed by patients, others think we have already gone too far in our procurement practice and are taking organs from people who are not yet dead. How can brain-dead patients on ventilators be described as dead, when the organism is in so many ways functioning as normal—even to the extent of being able (with intensive enough support) to complete gestation? It may be legitimate to switch off the ventilator and let such patients die, since doctors are allowed—indeed required—to discontinue treatment that is no longer of any benefit to the patient. But it is certainly not legitimate to kill them by mining them for their organs; and that, some people claim, is what we are already doing.

According to people who hold this view of things, then, a suspicious public is quite right to be afraid that the medical profession cannot be trusted to wait until we are dead before starting to collect organs. They are doing it all the time, and cheating the rest of us by shifting the official criteria for recognizing death. According to the critics, current standards allow people to be declared dead before they really are.

This looks like a serious matter. How, then, can the dispute between the two sides be resolved? Are these people on ventilators really dead or not?

The new problem of recognizing death

The problem looks real enough, but on the other hand there is something very puzzling about it. If we know so much more than we used to about the workings of the body, how can it be so much harder now to tell when someone is dead? It used to look as though the advance of science was making the matter easier. Once we understood the workings of the cardio-pulmonary system we could declare death, with confidence, at an earlier stage in the closing-down process than when we had to wait for coldness and stiffness to make sure. Now that we know even more, surely we should be able to say for certain even sooner. What is the problem?

The answer seems to be that even though the question is still expressed in the traditional way—as whether the person is really dead or not—the new problem is in fact *quite different* from the traditional one. The old problem was essentially about certainty: certainty that a non-responsive, apparently insensate body had reached a state of deterioration that was irreversible. To whatever extent people did not know enough about how the body worked and exactly what state it was in, they could not know whether it held any potential for return to recognizable life. Romeo got it wrong with Juliet; he thought she was dead when she was not. Cordelia looked dead, but Lear hoped that a feather might show that she was still alive. Modern technology could have shown them both exactly what the situation was.

However, the problem we confront now is a quite different one. We have advanced enormously in our abilities to detect what is going on in the body, and to predict the chances of restoring any lost function. We also know for certain that there is no chance whatever—in any foreseeable state of technology—of any restoration of a brain-dead person on a ventilator to conscious life or spontaneous breathing. But we have now separated, by means of the ventilator, the functioning of the crucial elements of life that used to function or fail pretty well together: heart, lungs, and brain. The brain stem has irreversibly gone, but the lungs and heart are still going. The question now is not *whether there is any chance that the person will come back*: we know the answer to that. The problem is no longer about certainty of irreversibility, but about *which elements* of the whole organism need to have gone irreversibly before the person is really dead. In other words, the problem now is not whether the departure is *permanent*, which was the old question, but whether it is *complete*. It is not whether we are certain that particular functions have irreversibly ceased, but *which* functions need to have ceased irreversibly for the patient to count as dead. This is a totally different question.

Another way of stressing the difference between these two questions is to consider the kind of investigation and analysis needed to answer them. One is a matter of technical expertise: a matter of whether some bodily failure is reversible, and to what extent. Doctors are (we hope) the experts in this matter. They know enough about the body to know about reversibility, and how much chance there is of it. They also know (again we hope) when prognosis is unreliable, which is itself an essential aspect of medical expertise. But *no amount of medical expertise* can answer the new question. The problem is not about the state the body is in, or prognosis for restoration of any aspects of its functioning. It is that we do not know what we should *count* as completing the death of the person. That is the nature of the disagreement between the people who now dispute whether the person is 'really dead'. If doctors can agree about which functions have irreversibly gone, while still disagreeing or remaining puzzled about whether the person as a whole should be counted as dead, what kind of argument or evidence could possibly resolve their disagreement?

This is another matter for thinking through by individual enquirers, because the way different people analyse the problem will depend on their underlying views—or assumptions—about the nature of the world in general and life in particular. However, it is useful, as a guide, to distinguish between two broadly different kinds of view about the nature of life and death.

Most cultures seem to have regarded the difference between the living and the non-living as consisting in the animation of matter by some extra element: some spirit, or soul, or life force, or whatever.

This is certainly an intuitively plausible idea. There is no obvious difference between a clearly living body and a newly dead one except the totally different ways in which they behave, so it is not unreasonable to suppose that what must account for it is the departure of some invisible entity that did the animating. According to this kind of view death must be the state the body is in when that extra element has completely gone. There are of course innumerable variations on this general theme, but the general idea tends to be that there is a soul of some kind, which, depending on the culture, may go off to heaven, hover around in a disembodied state perhaps tormenting the living, migrate into other animals or people, or unite with some kind of world soul.

According to views of this kind there is an objective truth about whether the brain-dead patient on the ventilator is alive or dead, since it is determined by whether the soul is still in residence or not. The problem is, however, that we have no way of telling. Our only evidence for the existence of the extra element is the way the body is behaving, and in this new situation we do not know how to interpret the evidence we have. Perhaps the soul is still there while the ventilator is keeping the body going, but perhaps it is not—and souls are not a kind of thing that can be detected by science. The answer would have to be discovered, if at all, by something like religious revelation—but religions have never (as far as I know) tried to do this. Religions have just relied on the same evidence for death as everybody else.

The difficulty of trying to identify some objective point of death is reinforced by the fact that irreversibility itself is not irreversible. Technology may eventually be able to reverse what could not be reversed before. When the cardio-pulmonary criterion of death was established it was true that once the heart had stopped there was no possibility of return. Cardiac cessation was final and therefore regarded as evidence of death. But in the 1960s, after a couple of centuries of effort, cardio-pulmonary resuscitation was discovered, and as a result there was a short time after the cessation of breathing and heartbeat in which it might be possible to start them again. Did that mean that in that short interval the soul had not actually gone, and that until the discovery of CPR we had been declaring death too soon?

If so, what happens if the cryonics people—the ones who offer to freeze you in the hope that when a cure is eventually found for whatever killed you, they will be able to thaw you out again and restore you to life—turn out to be right? Will that mean that until the point at which successful freezing is impossible in principle the person really is alive, complete with soul, and therefore that the frozen people are alive? According to the extra-ingredient view of life there is an objective truth about whether people in these strange conditions are alive or dead, and if we have been getting it wrong we may have buried or burnt millions of people alive. But it is something science will never be able to tell us.

Contrast that kind of view of the nature of life with the quite different one, increasingly accepted as the life sciences have developed, that life and consciousness are not the result of some extra element, but—however mysteriously—a function of the arrangement of material parts. Life gets going by the fusion of gametes, the splitting of cells and so on, and develops until in time the bits start coming apart and ceasing to function, and eventually the organism is dead.

Here the question of whether the person is really dead is quite different. When you know everything that is going on in the body, that does not provide evidence for the presence of some extra, immaterial entity pushing from behind the scenes. It means you know *all there is to know*. In contexts other than that of trying to identify a point of death there is nothing puzzling about describing the state of a body in this way. We can understand the idea that any function may begin to decline, or may stop altogether, and may be remediable (reversible) or substitutable so that the function resumes. That is the whole idea of transplants: an organ can totally cease to function but be replaced by a working replacement from somebody else. There can also be artificial replacements (hip joints), or machines to boost what is failing (pacemakers), or machines to take over completely the functions of organs that have failed (ventilators, dialysis machines). We can describe all this, and monitors can tell us all kinds of things about the body that we could not observe without them. They can even tell us what is going on in the brain. But the problem of identifying death is quite different. We know what a dead body is, and we know what a living body is; but when we are asked to pronounce on a body in a penumbral state, by saying what the characteristics are that determine whether it is alive or dead, we are puzzled because there seems to be no basis for a definitive answer, any more than to the question of when some borderline colour on a spectrum is really yellow or orange. If you take this second view of life and death, the problem is not that we cannot *tell* whether the person is alive or dead—not that we need more information—but that the question cannot be given a definitive answer at all.

In other words, the way you understand the question of whether the person on the ventilator is dead depends on your world view. If you take the extra-element (substance dualist) view of life, it has an objective answer; if, on the other hand, you think there is nothing more to life than a complex arrangement of material substances, the question of whether someone in one of these penumbral states is alive or dead has no definitive answer, and when you know all there is to know about the state of the body there is no further question to ask. The trouble is, however, that *either* way medical science cannot answer the question of whether the person is alive or dead, and that is what has plunged us into this new confusion. We have always taken the question of when death occurs as one to be settled by scientific expertise—essentially by the medical profession—and when it was a matter of establishing whether some physiological state should be regarded as definitely permanent, that was fine. But now the question is *which* permanent physiological states should *count* as death, and this is not a scientific question.

We seem to be in an impasse. We have strong moral and legal principles about not killing people or cutting them up before they are (definitely) dead, and we need to take transplant organs before they deteriorate through lack of oxygen when ventilation is discontinued, but we cannot answer the question of whether the prospective source of the organs is dead or not. One group does not know the answer, the other thinks the question as it stands has no definitive answer. There must also be many more people who automatically ask the question about whether the patient is dead, and presume there must be an objective answer, but are not even sure what the nature of any puzzlement is. They are just uneasy about what is going on when organs are taken from bodies that seem to show a great many signs of life. So where do we go from here?

A different kind of question

When a problem becomes intractable in this kind of way, it is usually a sign that it needs radical reformulation.

The pressing problem we have about patients in penumbral states is the practical one of how to *treat* them. Most people, apart from the minority who have started questioning the dead donor rule, take it for granted that people should not be treated as dead until they definitely are; and we have always relied on doctors to tell us when somebody has crossed the line between life and death. Now, however, they have told us all they can and we are still often puzzled about the practical question of when we are justified in treating people as dead. Perhaps, then, instead of trying to answer the unanswerable question of whether they are really alive or dead, we should start with the moral question of why it *matters* so much whether people in these marginal states are alive or dead. What, exactly, is bad about treating the living as if they were dead? If we can establish why it matters, that should help us to decide into which category of treatment anyone should come, and which risks to take in cases of doubt. In other words, we need to decide the *moral* question first, and then, in the light of that decision, work out what we need to know about the physical state of the body in order to make decisions about treatment.

There are various different possible answers to this moral question, but—as in the case of question of what death actually is—it is important in particular to distinguish between two radically different kinds. One view is that human life matters because it is intrinsically sacred: the 'sanctity of life' view. The other is that it matters essentially because it matters to the person who is living it. There are many variations of detail within each of these categories, and most people in practice probably hold a more or less confused combination of the two, but the differences between them are deep. Although their practical implications overlap in many contexts, there are many others in which they do not.

In its fully-fledged version, the sanctity-of-life idea is usually rooted in the belief that life matters because it belongs to God, and our duties to human life derive from our duty to God. Human life is valuable in itself, quite irrespective of its value to the person whose life it is or to anyone else, and duties are owed to human life as such. Of these the clearest is the negative duty of never ending innocent human life deliberately. Individuals also have positive duties to sustain lives for which they have responsibility, although these duties have their limits, which can be regarded as reached when 'extraordinary means' are required to keep life going. At that stage people may be allowed to die, even though the duty not to kill remains absolute. Respect for human life also requires its not being used merely as a means to other ends.

The other view about the value of human life is that it derives its essential and intrinsic (as opposed to instrumental) value from its value to the person living it. This means that we should think about the duties we owe the living in terms of what matters to and for living individuals themselves. The question of why we should not treat them as dead before they are should therefore be understood in these terms. (It may be worth considering, before reading further, why it matters to you personally that you are not treated as dead before you are.) One element of what matters seems to be the sheer value of our lives to us. Being treated as dead before we are is likely to result in our actually dying prematurely, and we will lose the chance of coming back from whatever state has been mistaken for death. We also think that being treated as dead when we are not must potentially be a terrifying experience. The horror of premature burial—the real fear of people who arranged to have bells in their graves just in case, or wanted their hearts removed or pickled before burial to make absolutely sure they were dead—would be an instance of both concerns.

This view of the value of life is quite different from the first, since the sanctity-of-life view has nothing directly to do with the interests of the person living it. If the duties to the living derive from duties to God, and are to human life as such, the implication is that (innocent) life must not be ended deliberately even when it is worse than nothing for the person living it. On that view euthanasia and suicide—self-murder—are as wrong as more familiar kinds of murder. If, in contrast, the value of life lies primarily in its value to the person living it, it ceases to have any intrinsic value when it has no value to that person, and has positive disvalue if it becomes worse than nothing. This view implies that there is nothing wrong in principle with suicide or with euthanasia—where 'euthanasia' is understood as death that is genuinely in the interests of the person who is to die.[‡]

Obviously the question of which kind of view—and which of the innumerable variations of them—is right is much too large to embark on here. All that is needed here is to point out that any enquirer into transplant ethics needs to come to some conclusion about the matter, and then consider what that view implies for the treatment of people in these new, technologically produced, penumbral states between clear life and clear death. In particular, they need to work out the implications of their own view for the moral status of brain-dead people on ventilators.

[‡] Hitler's 'euthanasia' programme was simply miscalled: the deaths were not for the benefit of the people dying. Nor is the killing of defective newborns euthanasia, except in cases where their lives are predicted to be worse than nothing.

For people who hold the person-centred view of the value of life, the principle of the matter is entirely clear. That view implies that all obligations to the living end with the final loss of consciousness. Nothing that could reasonably count as murder (wrongful killing) can occur beyond that point, because any residual life there may be in the organism has *no further value to the person who was alive,* and therefore no intrinsic value at all. For the same reason nothing that was done to preserve organs after that stage could be objected to on the grounds of treating a living person merely as a means to an end, since there is no longer any person who could have any grounds for objection to such treatment. Any reasonable objections beyond that point could only be of a kind that might be made to some treatment of the dead. If, therefore, the purpose of declaring death is to justify the recognition of a radical change of moral standing, this is the point at which it should be made. From the moral point of view, we should be able to declare death whenever scientists are able to declare with the necessary degree of certainty that consciousness has entirely and finally ended.[§] What happens after that point is just a residual closing down of the morally unimportant elements, to be regarded in the same way as the residual digestive processes after cardio-pulmonary death, or the continued growth of hair and fingernails.[5]

[§] This criterion leaves entirely open the scientific question of when this can in practice be done—a matter which, as with all such matters, can be expected to change in the light of scientific and technological advance. It is irrelevant to point out that there are difficulties about detecting consciousness, and that we have discovered evidence of it in some patients previously thought to be totally unconscious. The criterion implies that to whatever extent there may be doubt about unconsciousness or its permanence, death cannot appropriately be declared.

It is probably already obvious that this second view of why life matters, and when it should be regarded as having ended, is identical in practice with the view that we should start preserving and even taking organs when people's interests have finally gone, but before they are dead. Both views imply that terminal unconsciousness marks the appropriate end of the duties to the living: the difference between them is only one of terminology. One way of expressing the idea is that people should be *regarded as dead* when conscious life has ended; the other is that final loss of consciousness should mark the *change in moral treatment* that has traditionally gone with death, even though the human organism—the human being—is still alive. One account keeps the traditional account of how the dead should be treated, but recommends shifting the traditional basis on which death should be declared. The other keeps the traditional account of when death occurs—roughly, when the organism is no longer functioning as a whole—but recommends a change in moral views about how living people may be treated after consciousness has finally gone.

This demonstrates a serious practical problem faced by people who hold this person-centred view of why life matters, and want to persuade others to accept it. The difficulty is that the term 'death' has traditionally carried two quite distinct implications. One is that the organism has reached a particular kind of physical state; the other is that a change in moral standing has occurred. Because the two had always been presumed to go together there seemed no need to think in terms of more than one concept. As a result it was taken for granted that doctors, who were supposed to be able to tell us about the physical situation, would *in doing so* be giving the answer to the question about moral standing. But according to the person-centred view of why human life matters, the familiar moral and physical aspects of death may be drawn far apart. This means that either of the alternative descriptions just given will go against part of the way we have traditionally thought about death. One of them asks us to accept as dead people who still show many signs of being alive; the other asks us to treat admittedly living beings in ways that we have always regarded as appropriate only for the dead. It is not surprising, therefore, that it is difficult to make either of them seem intuitively acceptable. Against the background of our traditional ways of thinking, one implies the moral outrage of killing or cutting up the living, while the other involves describing people as dead when they seem obviously alive.

To meet this problem, some philosophers who accept this account of the value of life have adopted a way of describing the situation that amounts to accepting the 'twice dead' paradox, by saying that we should distinguish between the death of the *person* and the death of the human *organism*. This is of course in effect what the Harvard group was saying, and it does look as though something of the kind is needed. The simple 'dead or not?' question invites a misleading answer either way—which gives people who take an organism-centred sanctity-of-life view a political reason for wanting to keep to that way of thinking. For people who take the person-centred view of the value of life it is therefore probably essential to reject the old terminology. They need to insist on saying that different parts or aspects of the human being can die at different times, and that what we need to decide is the *moral* question of how we should treat human beings at different stages in the closing-down process. The world has been radically changed by science and technology, and we must not try to force our description of it into moral categories that seemed adequate when everything was different.

Still, questions about how to describe the situation are about policy, with all the complexities that involves, and here I am considering only principle. From the person-centred view of the value of life there is no problem at all about counting brain-dead people as dead. The problem is the other way round: that the law still does not recognize morally valuable life as having ended in the other cases of terminal unconsciousness.

What, then, about the implications of the sanctity-of-life view, which holds that our duties are to human life as such, irrespective of its value to the person whose life it is? This raises more of a problem, because the principle in itself gives no indication of when life should be taken to begin and end. People who accept this view of life usually seem to take for granted that there is a definite, objective beginning and end of each life—which is still widely thought of in terms of the presence or departure of a soul. Since there is no direct way of observing souls, the way the span of life is generally understood is shown in practice by the many people who hold what are now known as Pro-Life attitudes. The relevant entity is taken to be the human organism. So, for instance, as science gradually extended its understanding of how human life developed, the prohibition of killing was extended to apply to abortion at any stage, whereas earlier it had been prohibited by the Church only after 'ensoulment' had been regarded as taking place, at quickening.[6] And the prohibition of killing is also taken to apply in the case of marginal states at the other end of life, such as patients in persistent or permanent vegetative states, whose souls the Pope recently declared were still in residence.

It is intuitively obvious why early embryos and patients in PVS should be counted as living human beings, but intuition starts to run into trouble where technology takes over the functions of the organism, and this is the problem for people who take a sanctity-of-life view when it comes to brain-dead patients on ventilators. And, indeed, this problem is reflected in the disagreement about whether such patients are really dead. The disagreement here is not between people who take the two different approaches to the value of life, but *among* the ones who hold the sanctity-of-life view. At least, this is what seems to be indicated by the fact that although the brain-death criterion is challenged by some of them, it is now accepted in the United States without the kind of vociferous, politically critical opposition that is encountered by abortion and embryo research.

So, should people who hold the sanctity-of-life view accept the brain-death criterion for death? The problem is a serious one for transplantation, because obviously the answer has significant implications for the retrieval of organs. If the person is alive, but no longer able to benefit from ventilation, it may be acceptable to switch off the ventilator on grounds of futility; but then it will be necessary to wait for cardiac death before organ retrieval can begin, and by then both the quality and (probably) the number of transplantable organs will have been considerably reduced. If, on the other hand, the patient is dead, the organs can be retrieved while the ventilator is still going, and will do very much better from the point of view of transplantation. It matters a great deal to get the answer right.

If people who believe in the sanctity of human life are to accept that the brain-dead patients on ventilators are dead, but that people in other states of terminal unconsciousness are not, they need to be able to explain what the relevant difference is. They seem to be accepting the Harvard criterion for recognizing death, but apparently not the Harvard justification—because what the Harvard people implied by the term 'person' has obviously gone in the case of other kinds of terminal unconsciousness, such as extreme cases of PVS, and these are not counted as death. How, then, might the difference be justified?

Perhaps it may be said that many other functions are still continuing normally in PVS patients. But a great many normal functions (heartbeat, circulation, digestion, excretion) are still continuing in the case of the brain-dead person on the ventilator, so what could be the relevant difference between the two situations? The most intuitively plausible distinguishing element seems to be the matter of spontaneous breathing. The patient on the ventilator, it may seem, is not *really* breathing. The machine is just pumping air into the body and so allowing the heart to continue, but it is quite impossible that breathing could continue if the ventilator were stopped. In the case of PVS patients, on the other hand, and comatose patients who are not on ventilators, the breathing is unassisted. So is the idea that the brain-dead count as dead because their lives are dependent on machines, but for which they *would* certainly be dead?

However, this criterion will not do. As it stands, it implies that innumerable machine-dependent people who are very obviously alive should count as dead. The patients who are dependent on ventricular assist devices or dialysis, for instance, would be dead but for these technological props. So, even more strikingly, would the ones whose hearts have been replaced by external pumps while they are waiting in the hope of a transplant. People in these situations are getting themselves to dialysis centres and pushing their pumps around the wards while carrying on conversations, so they are certainly not dead. And, in fact, no matter how much of the working body we managed to replace by machines, it seems inconceivable that we would count the person as dead as long as consciousness remained. This shows that permanent lack of consciousness is a necessary condition of counting someone as dead, but that still leaves the problem of why it should not also be counted as sufficient.

Perhaps, then, it may be said, the point of death should be regarded as reached when there is certainty of terminal unconsciousness *plus* the inability of the rest of the body to keep going without mechanical assistance. That gets considerably closer to making the distinction in the required place, but it still does not work. In the first place, if machine dependency is not sufficient for death, and neither is terminal unconsciousness, what relevant difference can be made by the combining of the two? (Compare the moral innocuousness of unpaid organ donation, and of buying and selling, when the two are considered independently.) It is not enough to find *some* difference between the other cases of permanent unconsciousness and this one; if it is to provide a justification for making the dividing line between life and death it must be one recognizable independently of that decision. But anyway, even that would not make the distinction in the place that is currently accepted, since by that criterion someone who is both definitely dependent on a ventilator, and permanently unconscious but not brain-dead, should count as dead.

So, unless someone can find an acceptable criterion for making the distinction, it seems to me that nothing short of religious revelation could show that the brain-dead on ventilators were dead but that the mechanically maintained but permanently unconscious for other reasons were not. And furthermore, I should have thought that if the matter were even in *doubt*, people who take the sanctity-of-life view would think they should wait for certainty before treating someone as dead. That would presumably imply that the machine support could be discontinued as futile and of no benefit to the patient, but that organs should still not be procured until all the main activities of the organism have ceased. It seems to me that the critics may be right: that people who accept the sanctity-of-life view have no justification for counting brain-death as death—unless they are depending on religious revelation, in which case their criterion will be of no use to people of other religions or of none.

This problem needs to be confronted not just by people who hold explicit sanctity-of-life views, but by all legislatures who accept that there must be a clear line between life and death, and that brain-death offers an appropriate criterion. If there is nothing objectively relevant to distinguish it from machine-dependent permanent coma of other kinds, there is no reason for not counting those as death too. And if that is reasonable, why not the ones who are finally unconscious but still breathing?

The decisions we make have a great deal of significance for the possibility of saving other lives by transplants. Once again, we need to be sure that we have adequate justification for our dividing line between life and death, since every time we place a terminally unconscious potential donor on the side of life we deprive other people, who definitely are alive, of the continuing life they might have had.

Conflicting world-views

In their fully-fledged forms these approaches to the value of life are rooted in irreconcilably different world-views, and they have radically different implications for practice. Both, as normally interpreted, set high standards for the duties owed to other people, but their different ideas about the moral underpinning of those duties means that the sanctity-of-life view sees those duties as extending to situations in which, according to the person-centred view, the residual life of the unconscious organism has no intrinsic value at all.

In practice, of course, many—perhaps most—people's direct moral judgements about how we should act in particular situations are consistent with neither view, and are underpinned by no coherent set of values at all. That is also generally true of law, at least in countries where there is a separation of state and religion. In the liberal West the longest established laws and moral intuitions originate in religious ideas about the value of life, but they have been subject to continual erosion—to different degrees in different places—by various combinations of expediency, compassion, secularism, and common sense. The origins still show in the absolute prohibition of killing, except in the very few places where euthanasia is allowed, and the insistence that any treatment given must be entirely in the patient's own interests until (what is currently recognized as) death. But this view has been modified nearly everywhere in ways that press in the direction of the person-centred view of the value of life without actually reaching it. So, for instance, abortion may be allowed, but only under specified conditions; suicide may be decriminalized, but assisted suicide and euthanasia still forbidden; embryo research may be allowed, but only up to a very limited stage of development. And, as I have already argued, this is also what seems to have happened in the acceptance of brain-death, but not terminal unconsciousness in PVS or other kinds of coma, as a criterion for death *simpliciter*.

In practice, advocates of neither of the two views of what makes life intrinsically valuable have, in a liberal democracy, much immediate hope of getting laws that fully conform to their own view of things. What happens is that each takes whatever opportunity it can to nudge things in its own direction by trying to enlist the intuitions of people who have no coherent views of either kind. So people who really oppose abortion altogether may work on trying to get the allowable time limit reduced by claiming that technological advances allow for foetal viability at an earlier stage of development, or people who really think that euthanasia should be readily available make policy proposals hemmed round with restrictions because those are more likely to persuade the people who are not totally opposed on principle.

However, although this kind of piecemeal politics is probably inevitable and even in some ways desirable, there is another issue of principle that is worth making explicit. When there are people of radically different moral views in a single population, some decision needs to be made about how to deal with them. There is no neutral position to be taken here. It is logically impossible to let everyone follow their own moral principles in all respects, because those will often actually conflict, and inevitably whatever overarching arrangements satisfy the holders of some moral views will not satisfy others. This is a problem with which liberalism has always wrestled, but which everyone now faces. An enquirer trying to think through these issues needs to reach some kind of conclusion about this matter, as well as all the others. How should a society decide about when to treat people as dead, if there is such disagreement about the point at which this should be done?

If we consider the fully-fledged versions of the two views about the value of life, what is significant is that one of them sets the point at which intrinsically valuable life ends much further along the closing-down continuum than the other. The person-centred view holds that people are (relevantly) dead at a stage when the sanctity-of-life view regards them as still alive. Surely, then, it may seem, the law should accept the later point? No decent society can want people to be terrified that they are going to be treated as dead before they are, even if they are wrong in their beliefs about the physiology of what will happen; and, as the transplanters keep saying, even from the point of view of organ procurement it is crucial to keep people on side.

But it is important here to distinguish between two quite different kinds of issue. One is the belief many people still have that *their interests* do not end until the organism as a whole is totally dead; the other is the moral belief that the *duty to respect human life* is owed until the human organism as a whole is dead. These two kinds of belief are frequently held by the same people, and can support rather similar conclusions at the policy level, but they are quite different in their underpinning principles.

Most people probably still take it for granted that there is a definite, objective point of death, and they may also believe that until that time a person may still possibly come back to normal life ('while there's life there's hope'). If they are aware that there are contexts in which there is dispute about when we should count people as dead, they probably think of it as simply a disagreement about when—scientifically—that objective point can be known to have occurred. The complexity of sorting out the *ethics* of the new scientific and technological situation is nothing like widely enough understood—among clinicians any more than the medically untrained public—so the question of whether someone is dead is usually regarded as a straightforward question of fact. So if, as a matter of fact, many people still believe they have something to fear until they are 'really' dead (whatever they take that to mean), that is something that needs to be taken into account at the policy level by anyone of decent ethical standards. Even if you accept that we can, scientifically, sometimes establish that there is permanent unconsciousness before the organism as a whole is dead, and that nobody really has anything to fear if they are treated as dead when they reach that point because their interests as living beings have completely ended, you may still think we should wait for popular opinion to catch up before we adopt a *policy* that might alarm a great many people. You may think that there is no objection of principle to treating people as dead when science has established permanent lack of consciousness, but when it comes to making policy you will still want to take into account many other morally important matters, such as making sure that people are not afraid of hospitals.

However, the distinction that has been at issue in this section and the previous one is *not* the distinction between people with different factual beliefs about when we can be sure that our interests as living beings have finally ended. It is the distinction between different *moral* views about the nature of our duties to the living. As I have said, it is often hard to distinguish these issues in practice, because people who are afraid of premature diagnosis of the final ending of their interests will support the same kinds of policy as the ones who think that we have a duty to life until the organism as whole is dead. But they are quite distinct, as is shown, for instance, in the case of palliative care specialists who will administer

terminal sedation to suffering patients—to make them unconscious until death—but think it would be absolutely wrong to perform euthanasia. The doctors who take this view (who are usually
explicitly religious) think they have a duty to protect the interests
of the individuals to the extent of preventing their suffering as far
as they can, but that their duty to human life stretches further than
that. To someone with the person-centred view of the value of life
there is no moral difference between inducing terminal unconsciousness and actually practising euthanasia, since the effect from
the point of view of the patient is identical. To the person with
sanctity-of-life views the duty not to kill goes beyond the interests
of the individual. To that extent it is not a duty to the person, but
essentially, even if not always expressed that way, a religious duty.
From a secular point of view it is difficult to make any sense of the
idea that the residual life of a permanently unconscious person has
any intrinsic value.

If so, the question about the clash of principles at the deep, world-
view level should be considered from the point of view of democracies that separate religion and state. There is considerable variation
of detail in views about how such matters should be managed—and,
again, there is no neutral position—but as a broad principle it
seems to be accepted in liberal democracies that people should be
free to follow the requirements of their religion as long as these do
not encroach on rights that should be guaranteed to everyone, or
impose costs on the rest of the community. If an approach
along these lines is accepted, it has significant implications. It
seems to make it impossible to justify, as a ground-level principle,
a social obligation to treat people as having the rights of the
living after they have become terminally unconscious. Maintaining

as a fundamental principle the idea that individuals must retain the full rights of the living until the human *organism* has totally ceased to function amounts to demanding religiously based duties from everybody, including people who do not accept them. It also imposes high costs on the society as a whole, both in penumbral lives maintained and in transplant organs lost, by demanding duties that cannot be justified in non-religious terms.

This is a difficult point to get across in practice, because debates are usually focused on policy rather than underlying principle, and my claim here is only about principle. To go back to the earlier terminology, my claim is that a society that separates religion and state should not accept as a *constraint* on policy the principle that human rights should continue until the end of the life of the human organism, even though there might possibly turn out to be reasons in practice for making that the policy. But that will depend on what the reasons are—and this is why it is so important, in moral enquiry, to concentrate on questions of justification rather than simply on practical conclusions.

To illustrate this, imagine a society working on the basis of the principle that what matters is the interests of people (while leaving individuals free to do what they regard as their duty to God), and decides on that basis that there is a prima facie case for saying that duties to the living end at whatever point science establishes permanent lack of consciousness. Thus:

Our duties to others derive from their interests.

People have none of the interests of the living when they have become permanently unconscious.

Therefore we should be free to treat them as dead when they become permanently unconscious.

Someone who wants to defeat that argument needs to insert a 'But...' premise. One possibility might be something like this:

Our duties to others derive from their interests.

People have none of the interests of the living when they have become permanently unconscious.

But...   *Many people do not believe that their interests end then;*
            they are afraid that there may be a chance of their re-
            turning to life.

            Even though they are wrong, we should not adopt a policy
            that will leave them in a state of fear.

Therefore we should *not* be free to treat people as dead when they are permanently unconscious (but must wait until whenever people will in fact no longer be afraid).

That argument as it stands is valid. Whether we accept the conclusion will depend on such matters as whether we think it is true that people have these beliefs, and how much social effort we think should go into supporting the interests of people with false beliefs.

But what about this argument?

Our duties to others derive from their interests.

People have none of the interests of the living when they have become permanently unconscious.

But...   *Religious people believe we are not really dead until the*
            organism as a whole is dead.

They believe we owe a duty to the living until that point is reached.

Therefore we should *not* treat people as dead when they are permanently unconscious, *but only when the organism as a whole is dead.*

That argument as it stands is not valid, because people who think that we owe a duty to the living as a religious obligation do not think *their own interests* are compromised if other people treat them in ways that fail in those duties—at least, not according to any theology I have heard of. Even if you, as a patient, hold the religious view that life should be treated as sacred until the human organism is completely dead, it is not *you* that is harmed, or has any reason to fear harm, if you are treated by others as dead when your consciousness has finally gone. You may have theological concerns about dying in a state of grace, but there is not much you can do about that after you have permanently lost consciousness. What is wrong by sanctity-of-life standards, at that stage, is not *what is happening to you*, but what these other people are *doing*. You might fear for the immortal souls of any politicians and lawyers and doctors who say you should be treated as dead when there is still residual life in your body, but you would have nothing to fear for yourself. What is compromised is not your interests, but what you take to be other people's duty to God. That in turn implies that if a society accepts that no public resources should be spent on purely religious duties, it should not allow religious views to influence the question of when death should be declared.

However, it is no doubt obvious that the discussion so far amounts to no more than peeking under the lid of a bottomless can of worms, which I shall desist from opening any further here because the depths contain issues much further reaching than the problems of transplantation. For instance, as soon as you start detailed thinking about interests, you start to raise questions about people in the innumerable states between full personhood and total unconsciousness. This is an area I have quite deliberately avoided here, but it is of enormous and increasingly pressing importance in medical ethics as a whole.

More generally, it is worth commenting that the deep divide here between religious and secular ethics, rooted in their different world-views, is one that is to a large extent hidden in ordinary debate by the fuzziness of most moral and political argument. A great many *immediate* moral judgements are either explicitly religious or religious in origin, but are routinely rationalized in secular terms. It is only when the arguments are analysed in enough detail that the differences become clear. My own suspicion is that several of the other disputes in the area of transplantation have deep differences of world-view at their root, and it is certainly true of many other parts of bioethics. The more science and technology break down the traditional barriers that underpinned much simpler, traditional systems of ethics, the more these deep differences of moral view will need explicit policies to deal with them.

Trusting the profession

Finally, in the light of this discussion of death and dying, go back to its starting point at the beginning of the chapter: the issue of the public trust transplanters are so aware of needing, and which is at its most acute in these end of life contexts.

Consider the following case. A group of transplant professionals was discussing the problems of reassuring the public about the matter of death, well aware that there was often confusion and disquiet about whether patients in penumbral states were really dead—not only among families, but among practitioners themselves. What the group concluded was that clinicians needed to fix an absolutely clear 'operational definition' of death, that would allow them as individuals to feel complete confidence in pronouncing death, and the profession as a whole to speak with a clear, united voice that would reassure an anxious public.

The concern, in that context, was with the psychology of establishing trust; and perhaps this technique might often produce it—though presumably that would depend at least to some extent on which part of the public was concerned, and how much confidence could be inspired by individual doctors. However, once again, there is a radical difference between persuading people you are trustworthy and actually being so, and even between intending to be trustworthy and actually, objectively, being so. The real question that needs to be answered here is whether the public *ought* to trust an 'operational definition' of death agreed on, as it were behind closed doors, by the medical profession, and then used by that profession to present a united, confident, trust-establishing, public face. And, given the arguments of this chapter, the answer is that it should not—not because the profession is untrustworthy in any ordinary sense, but because this is a judgment that lies outside the range of medical competence.

Traditionally, deciding the criteria for establishing the certainty of death has been the job of doctors, and legally it still is. People are dead when the doctors say they are. Furthermore, as already discussed, this has until recently been entirely reasonable. Our traditional concern about establishing death was to make sure people were not treated as dead until there was no chance whatever of their returning; and, as medical knowledge advanced, doctors were the people best equipped to recognize when this point had been passed. That was what happened when an understanding of the cardio-pulmonary system allowed them to establish a point of no return at an earlier stage than was apparent on the basis of non-specialist experience. It might well seem, therefore, that when it was proposed that brain death should be regarded as constituting death itself, this was another case of the medical profession's applying its expertise in essentially the same way: that it had made new physiological discoveries, and that those enabled it to establish new criteria for recognizing when death had actually occurred.

In fact, however, as already explained, the two situations were quite different. The decision that brain death should count as sufficient for death *simpliciter* was not a response to any new discovery. The state of *coma dépassé* had been understood for a long time, and it was already well established that people in this state could never return to consciousness or spontaneous breathing again. The problem was not the empirical, scientific, question of whether the state was irreversible, but the moral question of whether the final departure of these aspects of life was enough for the purpose of *pronouncing* death, given that many of the elements of what had always been regarded as constituting life were still working as usual. The decision that brain death should count as death, against the background of a general acceptance that people should be treated as fully alive until they were pronounced dead, amounted therefore to a *moral* decision that people in this state were dead enough to be treated in ways traditionally limited to the dead.

Given how significant the moral distinction between life and death is taken to be—how utterly different in law and convention is the acceptable treatment on the two sides of the divide—this was a momentous decision. In context, given the moral background, it meant that you could now start taking organs for transplant from patients in this state. By default, however, if you did the same to people who were not yet brain-dead—even if they were known to be terminally unconscious for other reasons, and even if they were also machine-dependent—you would be guilty of at least grievous bodily harm and probably murder. This is a massive moral distinction to make between two situations that differ only slightly, and which—as I have already argued—is not obviously defensible on any understanding of the value of life. But whether or not making a life-and-death treatment divide at this point can be justified, it is certainly not a judgment that can be made on the basis of a simple application of new medical knowledge to entrenched, accepted, values.

In other words, this is not a matter to be settled by the medical profession—even in consultation with lawyers and other advisors. This is a totally new kind of question, about what rights we should all have if we fall into these penumbral states, at what cost to the rest of society. The costs of our current principles are considerable. Recognizing a firm divide between life and death, with full rights of the living until what is currently counted as death, involves accepting not only lost transplant opportunities and therefore lost lives (which I mention first only because this is the subject of the book), but also such extremely expensive matters as sustaining what remains of life rather than accelerating the closing down process ('killing'), and maintaining personal dignity throughout. It is therefore, like other questions about socially and legally instituted rights and duties, a matter for public debate and society as a whole. Of course it is impossible to debate these matters rationally without massive contribution from medical scientists, since they are the experts on the relevant physiology. In particular, most of us will want to know in detail how certain the profession can be about unconsciousness, and the probabilities of different kinds and degrees of recovery. But that makes the specialists relevant as expert witnesses, whose job is to make their knowledge accessible to the non-specialists. It is not to act as judge and jury.*

This is part of a much wider point about the position of the medical profession in matters of policy making. A great many policy decisions are still made, if not exactly behind medical closed doors, then at least with the profession as their main instigators and acknowledged experts. I make no claims about the extent of this; I have no doubt that it varies a good deal between different countries and among individual practitioners, so as usual I am not so much intending to describe a situation as to comment on how such an attitude should be regarded where it exists. But there is a good deal of evidence that doctors are widely regarded, both in the profession itself

---

* And, incidentally, a similar point applies to philosophical contributions to all these problems. The philosophical disentangling of questions is, as I hope I have demonstrated, an essential part of policy debates when advancing technology is taking us out of our moral depth, but it is nothing like enough for deciding what the all-things-considered conclusions about policy should be. That is why this book does not make any detailed policy recommendations. It makes what I hope is a substantial contribution to the organ-procurement debate, by arguing that various fixed ideas are, by all our normal standards, unjustified, and that they should be removed from their current position as *constraints* on policy debates. That, however, is very different from offering detailed answers to policy questions.

and by legislators, as all-purpose experts in medical matters, including medical policy. This shows, for instance, in the considerable extent to which principles of ethics and policy are formulated by explicitly medical bodies (as in the cases already mentioned here of the Declaration of Istanbul and the principles issued by the World Health Organization, but also many others), and also—though this is beginning to change—in the heavy preponderance of medical representation on government consultative bodies about such matters. It also shows in many comments of individuals. In a recent conference, for instance, one surgeon said 'we wouldn't have all these problems if the profession had regulated itself', thereby, presumably, intending to imply that it was appropriate for it to regulate itself. On the same occasion another surgeon, familiar with the world of medical politics, commented to me that there was no chance of getting legislative change until the profession had been persuaded that it was needed.

There are two things to say about this kind of attitude, to whatever extent it does prevail. First, the standards according to which medical practitioners should practise are not matters appropriately decided by the profession itself. Having a particular kind of knowledge and skill, such as medicine involves, does not entitle its practitioners to say how it should be used. If people are to be licensed or employed by society to practise the use of their skills, the way in which those skills are to be used is a matter for society as a whole. This is entirely obvious in the case of most professions: nobody would think that the police or the army should decide to what use their special expertise should be put, or that food safety and nutritional requirements should be matters for food producers. But it needs special emphasis in the case of medicine, because the profession seems to be regarded by many of its practitioners as different from others, in having been from its beginnings underpinned by timeless principles of ethics which practitioners absorb with their practical training. (Another recent comment from a doctor: 'If only all doctors would keep to the Hippocratic Oath there wouldn't be any problems of medical ethics'.) Except perhaps in the very broadest sense, that medicine is supposed to do good rather than harm, it is straightforwardly false that the values of the medical profession have been timeless; but even if were true, it would be irrelevant to the question of whether society should demand that those principles should change. Medical ethics, in the sense of the standards that should be upheld by the people licensed to practise medicine, is not a matter for the medical profession.

Of course specialist knowledge is always needed for showing how particular standards should be translated into practical decisions. At some point we have to stand back and let experts tell us the means by which to achieve the ends we regard as personally or morally important; the only way to avoid that is to become specialists ourselves. But that raises the second problem about treating the profession as all-purpose experts in these times of technological change. Medicine is an intensely practical subject, whose training involves learning a scientific and ethical framework within which practical problems can be addressed and solved. There is nothing in that training to equip practitioners to recognize and deal with the ways in which technology is actually changing the fundamental nature of the problems they face—as opposed to presenting them with more difficult versions of the traditional problems—or to engage in the conceptual unravelling needed for identifying and clarifying the new problems. Many individual doctors may of course have a natural aptitude for the relevant kind of analysis, and be able to recognize the problems for what they are; but that is true of other people as well. The skills involved are not among the skills of doctors *qua* doctors.

To say this is not to criticize the profession. Doctors, like the rest of us nearly all the time, automatically and necessarily try to slot the problems they encounter into existing frameworks, and unless they were inclined to do that they would not be much use as practitioners. Nobody wants to be in the hands of a doctor who is agonizing over complex questions about the fundamentals of ethics and metaphysics rather than getting on competently with the job in hand—even if at some point in the future it might turn out to have been the wrong job in the first place. Practical people must make judgements within their current frameworks. But what all this does mean is that even if the medical profession could be relied on to accept that it should not make new moral decisions, it may not be obvious when that stage has been reached. It is not at all *obvious* that the question of whether a brain-dead person on a ventilator is 'really dead' is a different kind of question from that of, say, whether someone who is unconscious after an accident is really dead. It is not obvious that what faces us now is not a scientific, technical problem about how to put into practice existing values about the appropriate treatment of the living and the dead, but a new moral question about how to treat people in these newly produced, or newly recognized, penumbral states between what is clearly full human life and what is clearly death.

Presumably nobody has much idea about the extent to which public anxieties about organ donation at the end of life are rooted in a natural fear of being in the hands of unknown others, and how much they represent a glimmering awareness that there are deep, new problems in these areas, and that we should not be trusting the medical profession to decide at what point it is morally appropriate to treat people as dead. But to whatever extent the second is true, the feeling is right. If we do trust the medical profession to decide when people should be treated as dead in these new cases, that is because we have not understood the nature of the problem we currently face. If they and politicians who rely on their advice think they should be trusted to do it, they have not understood the nature of the problem either. Treating the question as a matter of medical expertise perpetuates and entrenches the misconception that there must be an objective point of death that the medical profession can identify, and that when they have done this the answers to the moral questions are obvious. It also places a substantive moral decision in the wrong hands. The matter should be one for wider public debate, and this cannot happen until there is a much wider understanding of why there are difficulties in saying whether people in penumbral states are alive or dead, and the discussion engages with the fundamental question of why life matters. The situation has changed, and superficial debates about policy details cannot deal with it.

This matter of trying to deal with a radically new situation by fitting it into an existing framework also raises again, from a different point of view, the fundamental tension at the heart of the transplants issue: the fact that the organ needed to treat one patient must necessarily come from somebody else. I began by saying that there was, objectively speaking, a permanent competition between the people who needed organs and their advocates, and the rest of us, who had them. But while this may be true at the theoretical level, my impression at the end of these analyses is that in practice the situation is rather different. The people who need transplants turn out to be piggies-in-the-middle of the real competition, which is between the public at large and the medical establishment; and this competition, it seems to me, can best be understood in terms of a determination on the medical side to absorb transplantation smoothly into the existing framework.

The attitude of the public, as the possibilities for transplantation became widely understood, was of course in one way directly opposed to the interests of the people who needed transplants. If the public had responded by saying that of course their dead bodies should automatically be taken for use by the living, the situation would have been very different. But, as we know, the response in general was fiercely possessive, and there was wide insistence that organs should not be taken without at least implicit consent. However, this public response met with hardly any opposition. Governments not only took it for granted that all the protections of the living should remain intact, but moved to extend similar requirements to consent for use of the dead; and these moves met no resistance from the transplant community. Hardly anyone, except the hard-bitten philosophers mentioned earlier, thinks the state should impound bodies, and even the people who advocate systems of opting out rarely recommend the hard version. All this works against the interests of people who need transplants.

However, people's initial ideas about their natural rights over their own bodies seem to have been stronger this. Although the public succeeded with barely a struggle in erecting walls against unauthorized invasion, it is pretty clear that they took it for granted that their transferable parts were *theirs*: in effect possessions like any other—with rights not just against having them stolen, but to control their transference. That, at least, is what is implied by the presumption that they were entitled to sell them, or to make conditional donations; and *that* assumption did not work against the interests of the people who needed organs, because the only thing people can to do with transferable organs is make them available to others who need them. The curtailment of these supposed rights, which necessarily worked against the interests of people waiting for transplants, was instigated by the medical community itself. This is not to make any judgment about what the public at large would have said if it had been consulted; but this is in fact what happened, and it is significant in itself.

Why, then, did the transplant community try to prevent some organs' being made available, at the cost of lives unnecessarily lost? Many of justifications were offered, but these simply do not work; and that leaves the interesting question of the real *cause* of the opposition. This is an empirical question, but—as in the earlier questions about why people react with such horror to the idea of organ selling, and object to the use of their dead bodies—the patterns of reaction can be used to generate hypotheses. And it seems to me that it can all be best be understood in terms of attempts to absorb transplantation into the existing medical background without too much change to familiar practice, even if the result is that fewer organs are available.

Here I am speculating, but in line with the analysis so far. There seem to be two striking ways in which the new transferability has produced an unfamiliar, understandingly unwelcome situation from the point of view of the profession. First, there is the matter of procurement from the living. It is against all the traditions of medicine to inflict damage on a living patient except for the medical benefit of that patient, so procurement from the living is therefore, in itself, an intuitive anathema to most medical people. In the case of close friends and relatives, however, matters are more familiar: doctors are used to working with families who will make sacrifices of all kinds for people they love, and quite often in these situations the donation can even be seen as positively good for the donor, who may be in danger of losing someone very close. Living donation under these circumstances can fairly easily be absorbed into familiar traditions of medicine. Samaritan donors, however—who come out of nowhere and ask you to cut organs out of them, for who knows what motives—are much more alien; and the idea that people should be damaged deliberately in return for payment is quite appalling. The impulse to keep living donation between families and close friends is, from this point of view, entirely understandable.

Deceased donation also raises various kinds of unfamiliarity. From the point of view of the profession, organs are resources to be allocated in the same way as others, and in systems with universal provision of medical care this means they should be allocated according to some principle of impartiality. Any specifications about their destination made by the sources of the organs or their relatives, or any kind of reciprocity scheme, would inevitably interfere with whatever arrangements were normally made any existing scheme of allocation. It is not surprising that the natural reaction of the profession is to resist the appearance in the system of resources with strings attached, and to accept only the ones that can be treated like other resources.

It seems to me, in other words, that the response of the Authorities to the advent of transplantation has been effectively to push it into familiar shapes: to ban anything that does not fit the existing patterns of medical practice, perhaps with occasional stretches here and there, but essentially insisting that organs should be as much like other resources as possible. But that is the point. Organs are not like other medical resources—not because body parts are in some mystical way special (a familiar idea, frequently invoked to justify all kinds of preconceptions that defy other attempts at justification), but because they come from other people, and people have rights. The fundamental, new question at the root of transplantation, which seems never to be addressed directly, is what rights people should have over their own organs, both while they are alive and after they are dead. Maybe they should have none; maybe, perhaps, people now will insist on rights over their dead bodies, while more enlightened people in the future will agree that they should be used for the public good. But this is the fundamental question that should be addressed, and so far it has not been. From the outside, at least, it looks as though the public has built a defensive wall around its property, and the medical community another around its traditions, while people who need transplants die in the no-man's-land between them.

How this fundamental debate about rights over bodies, and the other fundamental debates about penumbral states and the value of life would turn out in public remains to be seen. My guess is that there would be some surprises. But the main point to emphasize here is that these debates are not mainly for the medical profession. In these times of radical change, we all need to understand and discuss what is going on. And one essential element of this, I would add in closing, is a much closer engagement of medicine with practical philosophy.

Conclusion: Why careless thought costs lives[**]

Everyone knows that how patients fare under medical treatment must depend heavily on the knowledge and skills of the practitioner. If what is happening and what is being done are not well enough understood, the treatment is likely to fail in spite of the best of intentions. Semmelweis and his colleagues at the Vienna Lying-In Hospi-

_____

[**] For everyone too young to recognize this allusion, it is to a series of Second World War cartoon posters with the caption 'Careless talk costs lives', warning citizens about the danger of spies. They are easily Googlable.

tal in the 1840s were seriously trying to understand and prevent the puerperal fever of which so many of their patients died, but it turned out that they themselves were killing their patients, by coming from the dissecting room to the wards without washing their hands. The Chinese physicians who gave the First Emperor mercury pills were doing their best to meet his demands for immortality. The medical science we now take for granted took a long time to reach its present state, and it is not much more than a hundred years since doctors and hospitals could be relied on to cure more patients than they killed. The medical profession now knows that medical science is not just something you learn from experts and then apply to your own practice. It is a constantly developing field, and one of the recognized duties of doctors is to keep up with research in their field, and make use of the best available evidence in treating their patients.

What is much less well understood is that what happens to patients depends as much on the values that underpin medical practice and policy as it does on the state of knowledge in the field.

Knowledge and skill, in medicine and everything else, are in themselves morally neutral. To the extent that you understand the workings of the world you can put that knowledge to all kinds of use, for good or ill. Medicine is traditionally underpinned by a broad intention to do good, not harm, but there are many different interpretations of what that amounts to. Practitioners' own moral views, and those expressed in the frameworks of law and professional ethics within which they work, determine whether and how the available knowledge is used, and can have as much effect on patients as the state of medical science and technology.

For instance, after the discovery of anaesthetics some medical practitioners thought it was wrong to administer them during childbirth, because in the Book of Genesis Eve had been told 'in sorrow shalt thou bring forth thy children', and that any ease of that suffering would be against the will of God. If you were a woman in the hands of a practitioner with those moral views, you would suffer as much as if anaesthetics had never been discovered. (The practice became respectable when Queen Victoria insisted on being given anaesthetics during the birth of her children.) If you are a woman in a country where the ethical principles of your government and medical profession rule out abortion, you are as unable to get a safe abortion as if techniques for safe abortions had never been developed. If a country's ethical views about individual freedom and parental rights mean that vaccination is not compulsory, and anti-vaccination views spread, controllable diseases start to spread again. Some people's moral views about contraception and condoms contribute to the spread of AIDS. And if our current moral views directly or indirectly make unavailable the organs that might have saved patients whose own organs have failed, those people will be as dead as if transplants had never been developed.

This is not to suggest we should not have principles and policies to control the acquisition of organs. Of course we should. But if saving life and restoring health matter, it does mean that we should think them through with considerable care, to check that any obstacles justify the cost in lives lost and suffering endured. And we should be particularly careful to do this in all contexts where technology has made radical changes in the world, because we now know how inclined we are to make direct and immediate moral judgements, and to rationalize them almost without thinking. When some new situation appears, our immediate impulse is usually to squeeze the new situation into the constraints of our existing moral system, which—whatever its original merits—was simply not designed to cope with the changes. One striking case of this, in the context of transplantation, comes in the continuing reluctance to recognize body parts as property, which they have effectively become; another is to maintain traditional ideas about the objectivity of a point of death and its moral implications. Thinking through the implications of these changes is a difficult job, but it needs to be done.

To think of medical ethics as a set of principles, let alone one that is timelessly fixed, is like thinking of science as the particular set of facts believed at a particular time. Ethics, like science, is an enquiry, and, like science, it is one in which progress can be made. There are deep philosophical problems about its foundations, and, even when clarification of moral arguments has reached its limits, disagreements between people will no doubt remain. However, we are a very long way from reaching that point. Most moral reasoning is full of quite objective mistakes—many of them immediately recognizable once they are pointed out. It is just that they are easily missed by people who have not learned to look for them.

It was only after Semmelweis had identified how puerperal fever was transmitted that he could recognize that he had, in fact, been killing his own patients. The First Emperor's physicians can never have realized what we now know their medications must have been doing to their patient. In the same way, we may never know the extent of suffering and death caused by ethical views that their advocates themselves would recognize as unjustified if they thought them through in enough detail. We have reason to believe that a good deal of it is happening, nevertheless.

Careless moral reasoning, like careless medical practice, really does cost lives.

NOTES

CHAPTER 1

1. John Harris, 'The Survival Lottery', *Philosophy* 50 (1975), 81–7.
2. Recounted in Jonathan Glover, *Causing Death and Saving Lives*. Harmondsworth: Penguin (1977), 212.

CHAPTER 2

1. Cases of this kind have arisen more than once. See e.g. D. Josefson, 'Prisoner Wants to Donate his Second Kidney', *BMJ* 318/7 (1999). The case described here came from my colleague Chris Rudge (see acknowledgements in the Preface), who was one of the surgeons who refused to operate—though not, I am glad to say, because he thought the potential donor did not understand his own interests, but because he as a doctor was unwilling to be responsible for causing such harm to a patient. The story has a happy ending: the mother, who had been dismissed as unsuitable as a donor, turned out to be suitable after all.
2. Extra-judicial comment by Edmund Davies LJ, cited in G. Dworkin, 'The Law Relating to Organ Transplantation in England', *MLR* 33 (1970).
3. e.g. *R v. Brown* [1993] 2 All ER 75.

4. The relevant law has now been replaced. The Human Tissue Authority now vets all living donors and recipients, not just unrelated ones.

5. As endorsed by the 63rd World Health Assembly in May 2010, in Resolution WHA 63.22. Payment is dealt with in Guiding Principle 5.

6. 'The Declaration of Istanbul on Organ Trafficking and Transplant Tourism', *Nephrol Dial Transplant* 23 (2008), 3375–80 doi: 10.1093/ndt/gfn553.

7. This happened in Britain in January 1989. The case was reported and discussed in all national newspapers between mid-January and early February, e.g. in *The Independent*, 18 January.

8. Council of the Transplantation Society (1985), 715–16.

9. John B. Dossetor and V. Manickavel, 'Commercialization: The Buying and Selling of Kidneys', in M. Kjellstrand and J. B. Dossetor, *Ethical Problems in Dialysis and Transplantation*. Dordrecht: Kluwer (1992), 61–71.

10. R. A. Sells, 'Resolving the Conflict in Traditional Ethics which Arises from our Demand for Organs', *Transplantation Proceedings* 25/6 (Dec. 1993), 2983–4.

11. Dossetor and Manickavel, 'Commercialization', 63. See also G. M. Abouna, M. M. Sabawi, M. S. A. Kumar, and M. Samhan, 'The Negative Impact of Paid Organ Donation', in W. Land and J. B. Dossetor, *Organ Replacement Therapy: Ethics, Justice, Commerce.* Berlin: Springer (1991), 164–72, p. 166: 'A truly voluntary and non-coerced consent is also unlikely... the desperate financial need of the donor is an obvious and clear economic coercion.'

12. Dossetor and Manickavel, 'Commercialization', 63.

13. R. A. Sells, 'Voluntarism of Consent', in Land and Dossetor, *Organ Replacement Therapy*, 18–24.

14. See WHO guidelines, commentary to Guiding Principle 5: 'Such payment conveys the idea that some persons lack dignity, that they are mere objects to be used by others.'

15. Declaration of Istanbul: 'Organ trafficking and transplant tourism violate the principles of equity, justice and respect for human dignity and should be prohibited.'

16. Although it is still true that there is a general 'no property in body parts' rule in almost all jurisdictions, including the UK, there are a few signs of a shift in attitude. See the recent case of *Yearworth* v. *North Bristol NHS Trust* [2009] EWCA C iv 37 (4 February 2009). I am grateful to David Price for drawing my attention to this case.

17. See e.g. Charles A. Erin and John Harris, 'An Ethical Market in Human Organs', *J Med Ethics* 29 (2003), 137–8.

18. '*Organ trafficking* is the recruitment, transport, transfer, harbouring or receipt of living or deceased persons or their organs by means of the threat or use of force or other forms of coercion, of abduction, of fraud, of deception, of the abuse of power or of a position of vulnerability, or of the giving to, or the receiving by, a third party of payments or benefits to achieve the transfer of control over the potential donor, for the purpose of exploitation by the removal of organs for transplantation.'

19. 'Travel for transplantation becomes *transplant tourism* if it involves organ trafficking and/or transplant commercialism or if the resources (organs, professionals and transplant centres) devoted to providing transplants to patients from outside a country undermine the country's ability to provide transplant services for its own population.'

20. '*Transplant commercialism* is a policy or practice in which an organ is treated as a commodity, including by being bought or sold or used for material gain.' But note here that the term 'commercialism', as normally used, is not the same as allowing payment. If a government health service offered payment to donors, because it would help the donors while also enormously helping the patients on dialysis, and saving money for the health service because dialysis is so expensive, there would be no *commerce* involved. Turning allowing payment into commerce is another rhetorical device.

21. 'Transplant tourism' is given a disjunctive definition of which one element is trafficking, so that is covered by the wrongness of trafficking. Another is travelling for services which undermines a country's ability to provide its own population's transplant needs, which I have no wish to dispute. But the definition also includes 'transplant commercialism', which means that that its objectionableness in that form depends on the objectionableness of transplant commercialism—payment for organs—itself. The Declaration needs therefore to offer a justification for regarding transplant commercialism as objectionable.

22. Dossetor and Manickavel, 'Commercialization', 66.

23. Abouna et al., 'The Negative Impact of Paid Organ Donation', 171.

24. WHO guidelines, commentary to Guiding Principle 5.

25. Ibid.

26. See e.g. Abouna et al., 'The Negative Impact of Paid Organ Donation', 167.

27. M. Broyer, 'Living Organ Donation: The Fight Against Commercialism', in Land and Dossetor, Organ Replacement Therapy, 197–9.

28. Robert Frank, On Choosing the Right Pond. Oxford: Oxford University Press (1985), ch. 10.

29. I discuss these points in rather more detail in Janet Radcliffe Richards, 'Nephrarious Goings On: Kidney Sales and Oral Arguments', J Med Philos 21/4 (Aug. 1996), 375–416.

30. See e.g. Erin and Harris, 'An Ethical Market in Human Organs', 137–8.

CHAPTER 3

1. John Stuart Mill, The Subjection of Women (1869; widely reprinted), 1.

2. John B. Dossetor and V. Manickavel, 'Commercialization: The Buying and Selling of Kidneys', in M. Kjellstrand and J. B. Dossetor, Ethical Problems in Dialysis and Transplantation. Dordrecht: Kluwer (1992), 61–71.

3. See Introduction, p. 11 n. † .

4. This is not meant to be a claim about all societies. For instance, Reddy claims that for many vendors a positive motive is given by the duties of Hindu ethics, and that respect and self-respect increase because of a duty done (K. C. Reddy, 'Organ Donation for Consideration', in W. Land and J. B. Dossetor, *Organ Replacement Therapy: Ethics, Justice, Commerce*. Berlin: Springer (1991), 173–80). This section is intended as a series of thought experiments for anyone who has these feelings.

5. Land and Dossetor, *Organ Replacement Therapy*, 231.

6. Dossetor and Manickavel, 'Commercialization', 68.

CHAPTER 4

1. The reference is to the retention of organs at Alder Hey hospital in the UK. Information is widely available.

2. Organ DonationTaskforce, *The Potential Impact for an Opt-out System of Organ Donation in the UK*, Second Report, 17 November 2008.

3. This was said in a television programme in which I was involved. Unfortunately I have no record of its details.

4. 'Even in death our organs are not for the PM to snatch' (Minette Marrin, *Sunday Times*, 16 November 2008).

5. Gerald Warner, *DailyTelegraph* blog, 14 November 2008. I am grateful to Professor Jonathan Montgomery for both this and the previous reference.

6. Department of Health, *An Investigation into Conditional Organ Donation*. London: DoH (2000).

7. For instance, this seems to be the position taken in the WHO guidelines: 'The allocation of organs, cells and tissues should be guided by clinical criteria and ethical norms, not financial or other considerations. Allocation rules, defined by appropriately constituted committees, should be equitable, externally justified, and transparent.'

8. DoH, *Investigation into Conditional Organ Donation*, 25. The policy has since been slightly revised to allow for donation between relatives.

9. See e.g. T. Swierstra, H. M. van de Bovenkamp, and M. J. Trappenburg, 'Forging a Fit between Technology and Morality: The Dutch Debate on Organ Transplants', *Technology in Society* 32 (2010), 55–64, p. 60.

10. See n. 8. It is interesting that this modification came about as a result of public indignation at a case when it was insisted that the organs of a dead young woman should be allocated impartially to the people at the top of the waiting list—even though her own mother was on the waiting list, and, indeed, had to give consent if the organs were to be used at all. There was no public demand for the 'unconditional donation' rule. That was entirely the result of official action.

CHAPTER 5

1. In the case of the Exeter Protocol it was argued that they might be harmed, because they might end up in PVS (persistent vegetative state). This has not happened to anyone so far, but as the experiment was stopped by law there is not enough evidence to show that it could not happen.

2. R. M. Taylor, 'Reexamining the Definition and Criteria of Death', *Seminars in Neurology* 17/3 (1997), 265–70; R. D. Truog, 'Is it Time to Abandon Brain Death?' *Hastings Center Report* 27/1 (1997), 29–37.

3. You could, of course, take a kidney without killing, but that is presumably counted as intervention not in the interests of the patient, so would be ruled out under the previous criterion.

4. Margaret Lock, *Twice Dead*. Berkeley: University of California Press (2002).

5. This has apparently been disproved recently, but it was believed for a long time.

6. According to a recent Catechism of the Catholic Church, 'Human life must be...protected absolutely from the moment of conception. From the first moment of his existence, a human being must be recognized as having the rights of a person...The first right of the human person is his life.'

INDEX